NURSING84 BOOKS™

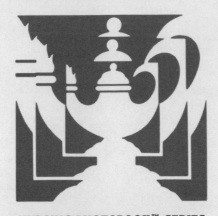

NURSING NOW™ SERIES
Shock
Hypertension
Drug Interactions
Cardiac Crises
Respiratory Emergencies
Pain
Neurologic Emergencies

NURSING PHOTOBOOK™ SERIES
Providing Respiratory Care
Managing I.V. Therapy
Dealing with Emergencies
Giving Medications
Assessing Your Patients
Using Monitors
Providing Early Mobility
Giving Cardiac Care
Performing GI Procedures
Implementing Urologic Procedures
Controlling Infection
Ensuring Intensive Care
Coping with Neurologic Disorders
Caring for Surgical Patients
Working with Orthopedic Patients
Nursing Pediatric Patients
Helping Geriatric Patients
Attending Ob/Gyn Patients
Aiding Ambulatory Patients
Carrying Out Special Procedures

Nursing84 DRUG HANDBOOK™

NURSE'S CLINICAL LIBRARY™
Cardiovascular Disorders
Respiratory Disorders
Endocrine Disorders
Neurologic Disorders
Renal and Urologic Disorders
Gastrointestinal Disorders

NEW NURSING SKILLBOOK™ SERIES
Giving Emergency Care Competently
Monitoring Fluid and Electrolytes Precisely
Assessing Vital Functions Accurately
Coping with Neurologic Problems Proficiently
Reading EKGs Correctly
Combatting Cardiovascular Diseases Skillfully
Nursing Critically Ill Patients Confidently
Dealing with Death and Dying
Managing Diabetics Properly

NURSE'S REFERENCE LIBRARY®
Diseases
Diagnostics
Drugs
Assessment
Procedures
Definitions
Practices
Emergencies

NURSING NOW™

RESPIRATORY EMERGENCIES

NURSING84 BOOKS™
SPRINGHOUSE CORPORATION
SPRINGHOUSE, PENNSYLVANIA

NURSING NOW™ SERIES

PROGRAM DIRECTOR
Jean Robinson

CLINICAL DIRECTOR
Barbara McVan, RN

ART DIRECTOR
John Hubbard

EDITORIAL MANAGER
Susan R. Williams

STAFF FOR THIS VOLUME

BOOK EDITOR
Kathy E. Goldberg

SENIOR EDITOR
Katherine W. Carey

EDITORS
**Holly A. Burdick
June F. Gomez
Patricia R. Urosevich**

CLINICAL EDITOR
Joan E. Mason, RN, EdM

DRUG INFORMATION MANAGER
Larry Neil Gever, RPh, PharmD

ASSOCIATE DESIGNER
Kathaleen Motak Singel

CONTRIBUTING DESIGNERS
**Lorraine Carbo
Darcy Feralio**

PRODUCTION COORDINATOR
Susan Powell-Mishler

COPY SUPERVISOR
David R. Moreau

COPY EDITORS
**Dale A. Brueggemann
Diane M. Labus
Jo Lennon
Doris Weinstock**

CONTRIBUTING COPY EDITORS
**Laura Dabundo
Timothy Gaul
Linda A. Johnson**

EDITORIAL ASSISTANTS
**Ellen Johnson
Suzanne J. Ramspacher**

ART PRODUCTION MANAGER
Robert Perry

ARTISTS
**Donald G. Knauss   Craig Siman
Robert S. Miele   Louise Stamper
Sandra Sanders   Robert Wieder**

TYPOGRAPHY MANAGER
David C. Kosten

TYPOGRAPHY ASSISTANTS
**Ethel Halle   Nancy Wirs
Diane Paluba**

SENIOR PRODUCTION MANAGER
Deborah C. Meiris

PRODUCTION MANAGER
Wilbur D. Davidson

PRODUCTION ASSISTANT
T.A. Landis

ILLUSTRATORS
**Michael Adams   Cynthia Mason
Jean Gardner   George Retseck
Robert Jackson   Brendan Riley
Robert Jones**

PHOTOGRAPHER
Paul A. Cohen

COVER PHOTO
Photographic Illustrations

**CLINICAL CONSULTANTS
FOR THIS VOLUME**

Paul M. Kirschenfeld, MD
Pulmonary Specialist, Atlantic
Pulmonary and Critical Care
Associates, Absecon, N.J.;
Attending Physician, Atlantic City
(N.J.) Medical Center, Shore
Memorial Hospital, Somers Point,
N.J.

Terri E. Weaver, MSN, RN, CS
Clinical Pulmonary Specialist,
Hospital of the University of
Pennsylvania; Clinical Instructor,
School of Nursing, University of
Pennsylvania, Philadelphia

NN5-011184

Library of Congress
Cataloging in Publication Data

Main entry under title:
Respiratory emergencies.

(Nursing now)
"Nursing84 books."
Includes bibliographies and index.
1. Respiratory disease nursing. 2. Emergency
nursing.   I. Series.   [DNLM:
1. Emergencies—nurses' instruction.
2. Respiratory Tract Diseases—nursing.
WY 163 R4337]
RC735.5.R467   1984   610.73'692   84-20306
ISBN 0-916730-80-8

CONTENTS

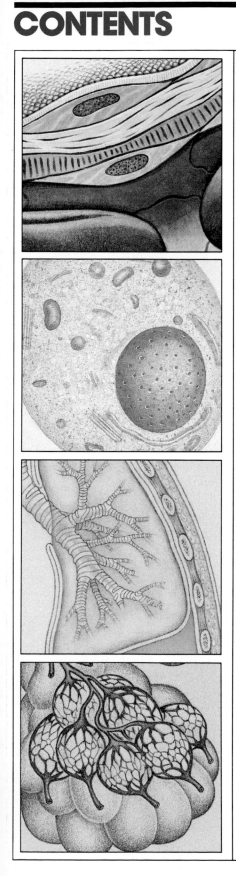

CONTRIBUTORS

At the time of publication, these contributors held the following positions:

Radene H. Chapman is an intensive care clinical nurse specialist and a research associate in the Pulmonary Division of LDS Hospital, Salt Lake City. She received her associate degree in nursing from Ricks College, Rexburg, Idaho; earned her BS from Brigham Young University, Provo, Utah; and received her MSN from the University of Utah, Salt Lake City. She is a member of the American Association of Critical-Care Nurses.

Barbara R. Ellis is an intensive care unit team leader at Genesee Hospital, Rochester, N.Y. She graduated from Genesee Hospital School of Nursing and received her associate degree in health sciences from Monroe Community College, also in Rochester. Ms. Ellis is a member of the American Association of Critical-Care Nurses.

Paul M. Kirschenfeld is a pulmonary specialist in private practice with the Atlantic Pulmonary and Critical Care Associates, Absecon, N.J., and attending physician at Atlantic City (N.J.) Medical Center and Shore Memorial Hospital, Somers Point, N.J. A graduate of the University of Alabama School of Medicine, Dr. Kirschenfeld is an associate of the American College of Physicians, an affiliate of the American College of Chest Physicians, and an associate of the American Thoracic Society.

Christine M. May is education coordinator of ambulatory services at Kettering (Ohio) Medical Center. Ms. May received her BSN from Ohio State University in Columbus and earned her MSN from Widener University, Chester, Pa., as a clinical nurse specialist in burns, emergency, and trauma. Ms. May is a member of the Emergency Department Nurses Association.

Carlene R. Peat, a pulmonary nurse specialist, is supervisor of the Respiratory Care Department at Kaiser Foundation Hospital in Walnut Creek, Calif. She graduated from St. Francis School of Nursing, Hamtramck, Mich.; received her BSN from Holy Names College, Oakland, Calif.; and received certification as a respiratory therapist from Pruitt College, Concord, Calif.

Paul C. Summerell is assistant head nurse of the Medical Intensive Care Unit at Duke University Medical Center, Durham, N.C. Mr. Summerell received his BSN from East Carolina University, Greenville, N.C. He is a member of the American Association of Critical-Care Nurses and of Sigma Theta Tau.

Laurie Burch Travers, productions and research manager for Vision Multimedia Communications, Inc., Oreland, Fla., produces audiovisual patient education programs for hospitals. She was formerly head nurse of the Medical Intensive Care Unit at Duke University Medical Center, Durham, N.C. Ms. Travers received her BSN from Florida State University, Tallahassee. She is a member of the American Association of Critical-Care Nurses and the Society of Critical Care Medicine.

Terri E. Weaver, an advisor for this book, is a pulmonary clinical nurse specialist at the Hospital of the University of Pennsylvania, Philadelphia, and clinical instructor at the University of Pennsylvania School of Nursing. She received her BSN from the University of Pittsburgh and her MSN from the University of Pennsylvania.

ANATOMY

RESPIRATORY CONTROL

MECHANICS

GAS EXCHANGE

ANATOMY

EXPLORING THE WHOLE AND ITS PARTS

The expanding scope of respiratory care demands a thorough knowledge of anatomy and physiology. After you identify a patient's respiratory crisis, you must apply your knowledge of respiratory basics to plan, implement, and evaluate your patient's care. To do this, you need to know what caused the emergency, which signs and symptoms to look for, and which complications could develop—and how to prevent them. The more you know about respiration, the more confident you'll be when caring for a patient in respiratory distress.

The hub of activity. The respiratory system is central to the functioning of most of the body's systems. When it performs effectively, it supports other body systems, contributing to the function of their organs. Likewise, an impaired respiratory system can cause failure in other body systems—sometimes causing organ failure that could result in death.

While the respiratory system contributes to the functioning of other organs, it depends on some of them as well. For example, the respiratory system needs the circulatory and nervous systems to be able to exchange carbon dioxide and oxygen in the lungs. When a person breathes, his lungs draw in oxygen from the air and distribute it to the blood, then remove carbon dioxide from the blood for expulsion into the air.

Besides performing this vital gas exchange cycle, the respiratory system helps maintain the body's acid-base balance to ensure a stable hydrogen ion concentration. Its other functions include warming the lungs' inhaled air and permitting speech by distributing air to the vocal cords.

And when another body system experiences a physiologic deficit, the respiratory system usually compensates. In a cardiovascular disorder, for example, the respiratory system works harder to supply more oxygen to the circulating blood.

Nonrespiratory functions. Some respiratory structures have important nonrespiratory functions. For example, the lungs:
• act as a reservoir for blood from the heart
• provide a minor excretion route for specific drugs and metabolites (for example, anesthetic vapors and gases)
• help inactivate the potent vasoconstrictor serotonin by taking it up in endothelial cells
• protect the heart, brain, and kidneys from emboli by filtering particles from venous system blood before it enters the systemic circulation
• help regulate water balance
• synthesize, release, activate, inactivate, and store chemical substances (such as prostaglandins, angiotensin I, bradykinin, norepinephrine, acetylcholine, histamine, and surfactant).

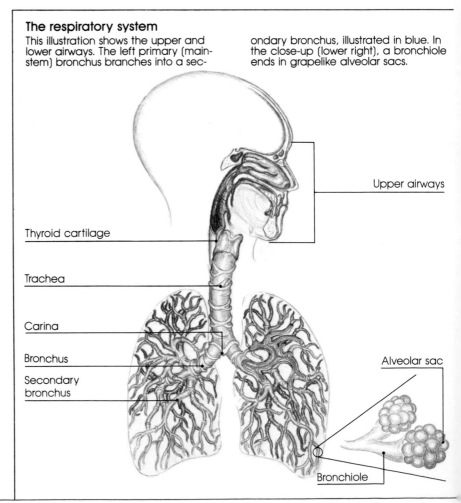

The respiratory system

This illustration shows the upper and lower airways. The left primary (mainstem) bronchus branches into a secondary bronchus, illustrated in blue. In the close-up (lower right), a bronchiole ends in grapelike alveolar sacs.

Upper airways

Thyroid cartilage

Trachea

Carina

Bronchus

Secondary bronchus

Alveolar sac

Bronchiole

A CLOSER LOOK AT THE UPPER AIRWAYS

What functions do the respiratory system's two major parts—upper airways and lower airways—play in respiration? The upper airways filter, warm, moisten, and conduct air to the lungs during inspiration and carry air away from the lungs during expiration. The lower airways facilitate the exchange of oxygen and carbon dioxide between the moist, internal alveolar surfaces and the tiny pulmonary capillaries surrounding the external alveolar wall.

Let's first review the five major parts of the upper airways.

Nose. During inspiration, air enters the body through the nostrils (nares), where small hairs (cilia) filter out dust and large particles. Divided at the midline by a septum, each nasal passage is formed anteriorly by cartilaginous walls and posteriorly by light, spongy bony structures known as conchae or turbinates.

Covered with a ciliated mucous layer, the conchae warm and humidify air before passing it through the nasopharynx. These tiny projections form eddies in the flowing air, forcing it to rebound in several different directions during its passage through the nose. This action traps finer particles, which the cilia then propel to the pharynx to be swallowed. If the air passage around the conchae is bypassed—for example, when a patient's on a ventilator—air must be humidified and heated outside the body. The conchae also divide nasal passages into the superior, middle, and inferior meatuses.

Sinuses. Four paranasal sinuses drain through the meatuses near the conchae. The maxillary and frontal sinuses are large mucus-covered, air-filled cavities; the sphenoidal and ethmoidal sinuses—also mucus-coated—consist of several small spaces in the nasal cavity's bony posterior portion.

Nasopharynx. Air flows from the nasal cavity through the conchae—which remain constantly open—into the nasopharynx. Within this structure are the pharyngeal tonsils and the eustachian tube openings, nestled in the lateral walls above the soft palate. (The eustachian tubes regulate middle ear pressure during swallowing and yawning.)

Pharynx. The mouth's posterior wall, the oropharynx, joins the nasopharynx to the laryngopharynx. Extending to the esophagus, the laryngopharynx is the lowest pharyngeal region.

Larynx. From the laryngopharynx, air moves into the larynx, which links the pharynx to the trachea. Two of its nine cartilages—the large, shield-shaped thyroid cartilage (Adam's apple) and the cricoid cartilage just below it—can be palpated in the neck.

The epiglottis, a leaf-shaped, flexible cartilage, hangs over the larynx. Its most important function is preventing food or liquid from entering the airways. The epiglottis snaps shut during swallowing, routing food to the esophagus. But it opens to allow air to enter the trachea and lungs.

The larynx aids in coughing, an important protective mechanism. When dust, dirt, or other irritants stimulate laryngeal sensory receptors, the abdominal and thoracic muscles contract, pushing against the diaphragm and increasing pressure within the tracheobronchial tree. The vocal cords open suddenly in a cough, forcing air and foreign particles out of the lungs.

The upper airways
Air enters the body through the nostrils, then descends through the upper airways, where it's filtered, warmed, and moistened.

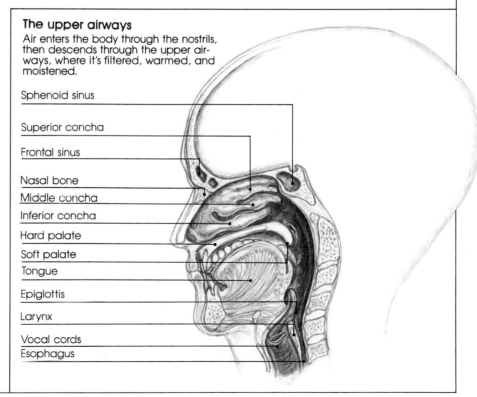

Sphenoid sinus

Superior concha

Frontal sinus

Nasal bone

Middle concha

Inferior concha

Hard palate

Soft palate

Tongue

Epiglottis

Larynx

Vocal cords

Esophagus

ANATOMY CONTINUED

TRACING THE LOWER AIRWAYS

The lower airways contain two portions: the conducting airways and the respiratory airways. The conducting airways—the trachea, primary bronchi, lobar and segmental bronchi—resemble an inverted tree. Their walls consist of cartilage, smooth muscle, connective tissue, epithelium, and nerves. Although the conducting airways dilate, constrict, and secrete and propel mucus in response to stimuli, they don't participate in gas exchange.

The conducting airways begin at the trachea. A tubular structure also known as the windpipe, the trachea extends about 5" (12.7 cm) from the cricoid cartilage to the carina, situated at the sixth or seventh thoracic level.

C-shaped cartilage rings with posterior openings reinforce and protect the trachea, preventing its collapse.

Bronchi. The trachea branches into two primary (mainstem) bronchi at the carina. The right primary bronchus, a more direct passageway from the trachea, is wider and about 1" (2.5 cm) shorter than the left primary bronchus. As a result, aspirated particles entering the trachea—or a malpositioned endotracheal tube—are more likely to drop into the right bronchus than the left. Like the trachea, the bronchi are lined with a ciliated mucous layer and reinforced with cartilage rings.

The left primary bronchus is about twice the length of its coun-terpart, and for good reason. Before branching into smaller bronchi in the upper and lower lung lobes, it passes under the aortic arch to the esophagus, thoracic duct, and descending aorta.

From here, the primary bronchi divide into secondary (lobar) branches. Accompanied by blood vessels, nerves, and lymphatics, they enter the lungs at the hilum. Each of the five secondary bronchi (right upper, middle, and lower, and left upper and lower) passes into its own lung lobe.

Bronchioles. Continuing to subdivide, these branches form terminal bronchioles, which supply air to the 18 lobules, or bronchopulmonary segments. As terminal bronchioles continue to branch, cartilage thins out and smooth muscle accumulates, narrowing the airways to an average diameter of 0.5 mm.

These tiny airways, known as respiratory bronchioles, supply air to the lobules. They also mark the end of the conducting airways and the start of the respiratory airways.

Alveoli. Once inside a lobule, respiratory bronchioles branch into smaller bronchioles, feeding into air sacs, or alveoli, at sites along the alveolar wall. Respiratory bronchioles end at alveolar sacs—clusters of alveoli.

Alveoli consist of Type I and Type II epithelial cells. Thin, flat squamous Type I cells, the most abundant, form the alveolar walls. Type II cells aid gas exchange by producing surfactant, a lipid-type substance that prevents total alveolar collapse. Alveolar cells, a small interstitial space, capillary basement membrane, and endothelial cells in the capillary wall collectively make up the respiratory membrane, where gas exchange occurs.

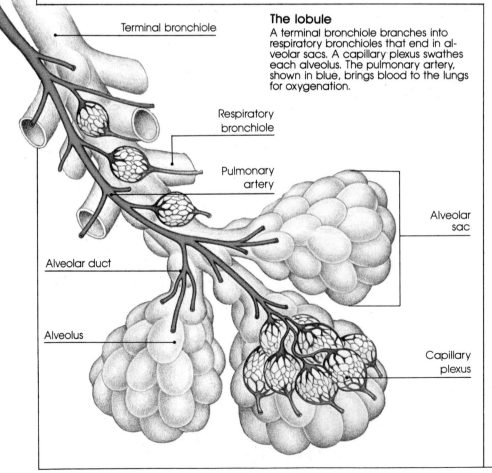

Terminal bronchiole

Respiratory bronchiole

Pulmonary artery

Alveolar duct

Alveolus

Alveolar sac

Capillary plexus

The lobule

A terminal bronchiole branches into respiratory bronchioles that end in alveolar sacs. A capillary plexus swathes each alveolus. The pulmonary artery, shown in blue, brings blood to the lungs for oxygenation.

THE LUNGS: RESPIRATION'S KEY

The most essential parts of the respiratory system—the lungs— are cone-shaped, spongy organs. Each lung has an apex, base, three borders, and two surfaces. The chest wall forms the lateral boundary for both lungs. The rounded apex of each extends about 1½" (3.8 cm) above the first rib; the broad, concave base rests on the diaphragm's convex surface. Along with the diaphragm, each lung base moves up during expiration and down during inspiration.

Fissures partially divide each lung into lobes—three lobes for the larger right lung, two for the left. The left lung's medial anterior surface wraps around and under the heart, forming a tonguelike structure known as the *lingula pulmonis sinistri.* The diaphragm separates the inferior surfaces of both lower lobes from the abdominal viscera.

Pleura. The visceral pleura, a tough, elastic-like membrane, envelops each lung and separates it from mediastinal structures, such as the heart and its great vessels, the trachea, the esophagus, and the bronchi. A similar membrane, the parietal pleura, lines the chest wall's inner surface and the diaphragm's upper surface, then doubles back around the mediastinum. At the hilum, the parietal and visceral pleurae meet, forming a narrow fold known as the pulmonary ligament. Both the visceral and parietal pleurae contain connective and epithelial tissues and a single layer of secreting epithelium.

An airtight region between the membranes, the pleural space can be seen only when air or water collects in it, such as in pneumothorax or pleural effusion. A thin film of serous fluid fills the pleural space, minimizing friction between the membranes during respiration and creating a cohesive force that makes the lungs move in synchrony with the chest wall.

The thoracic cavity. Some of the body's vital organs and structures are housed in the thoracic cavity, which is bound anteriorly by the sternum and costal cartilages and posteriorly by the ribs and thoracic vertebrae. Protecting internal thoracic organs, it also supports the chest wall, allowing the wall to move during respiration.

Mediastinum. A part of the thoracic cavity, this space between the lungs is enveloped by a thick extension of thoracic fascia. Extending from the sternum to the vertebral column, the mediastinum houses the heart and pericardium; thoracic aorta; pulmonary artery and veins; vena cavae and azygos veins; thymus, lymph nodes, and vessels; trachea, esophagus, and thoracic duct; and vagus, cardiac, and phrenic nerves.

The lungs in relation to other chest structures

The lungs occupy most of the thoracic cavity. Note the heart (outlined in blue) projected over the sternum and left lung.

- Clavicle
- Sternum
- Rib
- Trachea
- Lung
- Heart

ANATOMY CONTINUED

PULMONARY CIRCULATION: VEHICLE FOR GAS EXCHANGE

To achieve gas exchange, a network of blood vessels transports oxygen and carbon dioxide between the tissues and lungs. As you can see in the illustration below, four main arteries supply blood to the lungs: two pulmonary arteries and two bronchial arteries.

The pulmonary arteries originate from the heart's right side. Blood reaches the pulmonary trunk from the heart's right ventricle. The trunk branches into right and left pulmonary arteries, which continue to subdivide as they follow the bronchial airways through the lungs. Eventually, pulmonary arteries branch into microscopic structures called arterioles and venules, which enter the lung lobules and form capillary beds around the alveoli.

Gas exchange occurs at the alveolocapillary membrane, where the pulmonary capillary and alveolus meet. Oxygen diffuses into blood across the membrane, while carbon dioxide diffuses from capillary blood into the alveolus. Fortified with oxygen, blood flows through a branch of the pulmonary vein toward the heart. When it reaches the left ventricle, it's pumped through the systemic circulation to deliver life-sustaining oxygen to tissue cells and remove waste products from them.

The bronchial arteries, descending from the aorta and its branches, supply oxygen-rich blood to the conducting airways and pleurae. Because they're part of the systemic circulation, they play no part in the oxygenation of blood.

A concentrated network of lymph vessels drains the pulmonary pleurae and the highly elastic connective tissue surrounding the bronchi, respiratory bronchioles, pulmonary arteries, and veins. Lymph travels to collecting trunks, which route it to bronchopulmonary nodes at the hilum.

The lungs hold about 450 ml of blood—9% of the circulatory system's total blood volume. Approximately 380 ml fill the pulmonary veins and arteries; pulmonary capillaries hold the remaining 70 ml.

How pulmonary and systemic circulation interact

A network of blood vessels routes unoxygenated blood (shown in blue) to the lungs for gas exchange. The blood, now oxygenated, flows through the pulmonary vein to the heart, which pumps it throughout the body.

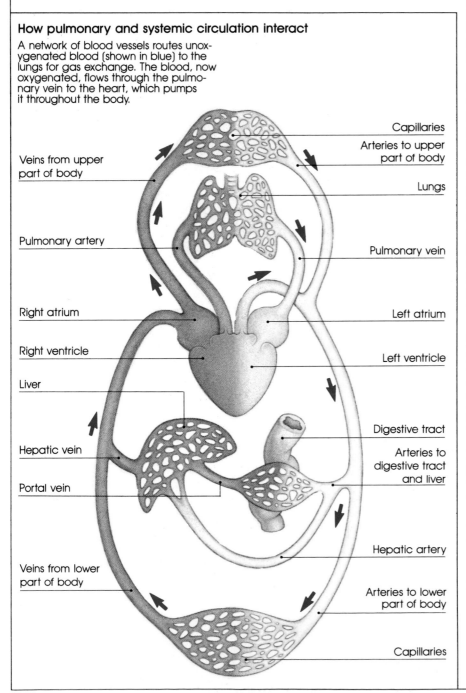

- Veins from upper part of body
- Pulmonary artery
- Right atrium
- Right ventricle
- Liver
- Hepatic vein
- Portal vein
- Veins from lower part of body
- Capillaries
- Arteries to upper part of body
- Lungs
- Pulmonary vein
- Left atrium
- Left ventricle
- Digestive tract
- Arteries to digestive tract and liver
- Hepatic artery
- Arteries to lower part of body
- Capillaries

RESPIRATORY CONTROL

THE BRAIN'S ROLE

A largely automatic, involuntary process, respiration's regulated by the brain and nerves, with help from certain chemical and physiologic factors. Even during respiratory distress, the nervous system adjusts the ventilatory rate to the body's demands so precisely that the blood's oxygen and carbon dioxide levels barely change.

Medulla. Home base for the mechanical control of respiration is the medulla oblongata, located inside the brain stem just above the spinal cord. Known as the body's respiratory center, the medulla oblongata controls breathing in addition to other respiratory reflexes, such as gagging, coughing, swallowing, and articulating. Most activity associated with breathing occurs in a site within the medulla called the medullary respiratory center. In this area, neurons associated with inspiration interact with neurons associated with expiration to regulate respiratory rate and depth.

However, these neurons also react to other impulses, particularly those from the pons.

Pons. Also located within the brain stem, between the midbrain and medulla oblongata, the pons contains two groups of neurons which regulate respiratory rhythm. To do this, they harmonize the transition from inspiration to expiration, and back, by interacting with the medullary regulatory centers. During this process, the apneustic center of the pons triggers inspiratory neurons in the medulla to stimulate inspiration. But these inspiratory neurons go one step farther to stimulate the pons pneumotaxic center, to begin expiration. They inhibit the apneustic center and stimulate the medulla's expiration neurons. Simply speaking, then, the pons paces respiration by

regulating rhythm, while the medulla controls rate and depth.

Nerves. The phrenic nerves from the third to the fifth cervical vertebrae innervate the diaphragm. Intercostal nerves innervate the intercostal muscles. Vagus nerve branches innervate the larynx. Although visceral sensation through these vagal fibers is, for the most part, limited to stretch, some vagal and sympathetic fibers are motor fibers of the bronchial tree's smooth muscle. Sympathetic fibers regulate vasoconstriction of the pulmonary arterioles.

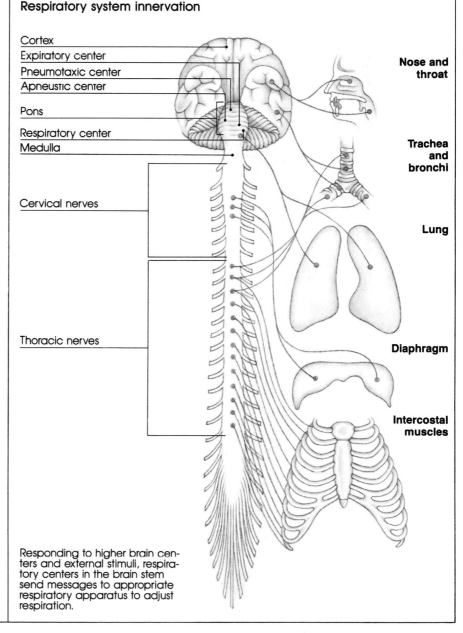

Respiratory system innervation

Cortex
Expiratory center
Pneumotaxic center
Apneustic center
Pons
Respiratory center
Medulla
Cervical nerves
Thoracic nerves

Nose and throat
Trachea and bronchi
Lung
Diaphragm
Intercostal muscles

Responding to higher brain centers and external stimuli, respiratory centers in the brain stem send messages to appropriate respiratory apparatus to adjust respiration.

RESPIRATORY CONTROL CONTINUED

HOW HERING-BREUER REFLEXES HELP CONTROL RESPIRATION

Physiologic factors such as lung expansibility (compliance), airway size, and resistance to flow also affect respiration.

When the lungs expand, they stimulate stretch receptors in the alveolar ducts, sending a stream of impulses along afferent fibers of the vagus nerves to the brain's respiratory centers. These impulses inhibit the inspiratory center, which then stops sending expansion signals to the diaphragm and external intercostal muscles. These muscles stop expanding, and expiration begins.

Conversely, afferent impulses responding to lung deflation inhibit expiration and bring on inspiration. Reacting to inhibitory as well as excitatory impulses, these reflexes, known as the Hering-Breuer reflexes, (after the men who first described them), maintain respiratory rhythm and prevent alveolar overdistention when the volume of inspired air exceeds 1 liter. However, Hering-Breuer reflexes may not be active in the adult during normal quiet breathing.

When the normal nerve passageway is blocked, Hering-Breuer reflexes carry on a secondary mechanism independent of the vagus nerve. A severed vagus nerve, for example, triggers prolonged and deep inspirations. In time, however, action of the Hering-Breuer reflexes stops the inspiratory center from sending expansion messages, and expiration begins.

THE RATE AND DEPTH REGULATORS: CHEMORECEPTORS

Chemoreceptors monitor the body's ventilatory status and signal respiratory centers to increase or decrease respiratory rate and depth. They respond to changes in carbon dioxide levels, oxygen levels, and pH.

In the anterior medulla, central chemoreceptors are particularly sensitive to alterations in the blood's carbon dioxide level and acid-base balance. Consider what happens when a person exercises, increasing his metabolic rate: the blood's carbon dioxide level rises. The carbon dioxide gas diffuses easily from the cerebral capillaries into the cerebrospinal fluid, which surrounds the central nervous system, interacting with water to form carbonic acid and to yield hydrogen ions.

Alert to the rising acidity, chemoreceptors stimulate the respiratory center to increase respiratory rate and depth. This action causes the person to hyperventilate. Sensitive to changes in the oxygen level, the peripheral chemoreceptors (located in the aortic and carotid bodies) alter the respiratory rate and depth in response to decreased arterial oxygen levels, or hypoxemia.

If the carbon dioxide level falls below normal, the central chemoreceptors slow breathing until cellular metabolism produces more carbon dioxide.

BLOOD PRESSURE'S ROLE IN RESPIRATION

Baroreceptors, spray-type nerve endings embedded in the walls of the aortic and carotid sinuses, also initiate respiratory changes when stimulated. Sensitive to pressure, baroreceptors react to sudden, sharp variations in blood pressure by stimulating a central reflex mechanism that allows for physiologic adjustments via vasodilation or vasoconstriction. For example, a sudden rise in blood pressure stimulates baroreceptors to send impulses to the brain's respiratory centers. These impulses inhibit respiratory activity and temporarily make respiration slower and shallower.

When severe hemorrhage triggers a sudden blood pressure drop, baroreceptor impulses slow down to quicken respiratory rate and depth.

CONTROLLING RESPIRATION CONSCIOUSLY

Respiration can be controlled consciously—for a short time—through nerve impulses from the motor area of the cerebral cortex. This enables a person to increase or decrease his respiratory rate for such activities as speaking, singing, or swimming. He could hyperventilate or hypoventilate long enough to seriously alter the blood's oxygen and carbon dioxide levels.

But conscious respiratory control can be only temporary, because the blood's carbon dioxide level is a stronger regulator of respiration than cortical impulses. Consequently, holding the breath increases the carbon dioxide level, since carbon dioxide isn't being removed by exhalation. As carbon dioxide levels rise, the inspiratory center relays impulses to the respiratory muscle to resume respiration.

MECHANICS

OTHER PHYSIOLOGIC FACTORS

In addition to lung inflation and changes in blood pressure and blood gas levels, other physiologic factors, such as temperature changes, airway irritation, and sensory stimulation, also affect respiration. Here's how: Nerve networks surrounding the bronchial and arterial trees contain vagal and sympathetic efferent nerves and vagal afferent nerves. When stimulated, vagal efferent nerves produce bronchoconstriction; sympathetic efferent nerves induce vasoconstriction; and vagal afferent nerves precipitate hyperventilation, coughing, bronchoconstriction and Hering-Breuer reflexes.

Irritants. Consider what happens when irritating gases, smoke, dust, or histamine stimulate irritant receptors in the mucous membrane lining the respiratory tract. Vagal afferent nerves carry the impulses to the respiratory centers, which in turn produce a sneeze to expel the nasal irritant or a cough or bronchoconstriction to expel the laryngeal or tracheal irritant.

Temperature changes. When blood temperature suddenly rises, such as from fever or exertion, the respiratory center increases respiratory rate and depth. Conversely, a drop in temperature, such as from hypothermia, temporarily decreases respiratory rate and depth.

Sensory stimulation. Sudden heat or cold, or an alarming sound or sight, may stimulate several receptors simultaneously. You may experience a temporary reflex reaction, for example, a gasp, respiratory rate increase, or momentary apnea.

Working together in perfect harmony, these factors supply the lungs with continuous airflow.

VENTILATION: AN INSIDE LOOK

We explained earlier how chemical, neurologic, and physiologic controls regulate respiration. But what about respiratory mechanics—the sequence of events that produces breathing?

Ventilation, the technical term for breathing, has two phases: inspiration, requiring muscle contraction and known as the active phase of ventilation, and expiration, the passive phase, which takes place as the muscles relax.

Ventilation occurs about 12 times a minute—more during strenuous exercise. Each breath draws about 500 ml of air into the lungs, continually replenishing them with fresh air while helping to rid them of waste products.

The lungs expand and contract in two ways: by movements of the diaphragm and by movements of the intercostal and other chest muscles. In normal, relaxed breathing (quiet inspiration), the diaphragm does nearly all the work. Stretching downward to contract, it pulls the lower lung surfaces with it, lengthening the chest cavity and inflating the lungs. During expiration, the diaphragm relaxes, and the elastic recoil of the lungs, chest wall, and abdominal structures compresses the lungs.

But what happens when breathing's not relaxed? How does the runner catch his breath at the end of a race? To meet his body's increased oxygen needs, he begins to pant, calling chest muscles into play. In this type of breathing, known as costal breathing, movements of the chest muscles account for more than half of lung expansion. As the runner breathes in, the abdominal and internal intercostal muscles contract, lifting the rib cage and sternum to allow the lungs to expand. As he exhales, these muscles contract, pulling the lower ribs down to compress the lungs. Unlike diaphragmatic breathing, costal breathing is shallow and rapid, and expiration's active rather than passive.

Lung expansion and contraction

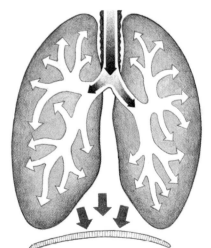

Inspiration: Stretching downward, the diaphragm contracts and the chest cavity enlarges, inflating the lungs.

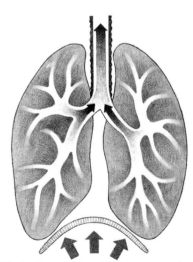

Expiration: As the diaphragm recoils, the chest cavity shrinks, compressing the lungs.

MECHANICS CONTINUED

PRESSURE GRADIENTS: THE FORCE BEHIND AIR MOVEMENT

What makes air move in and out of the lungs? Pressure gradients—differences in pressure from one location to the next. A fluid always moves *with*, not against, the pressure gradient, traveling from an area of higher pressure to one of lower pressure.

The chest movements you just read about establish pressure gradients in the respiratory tract. These movements produce pressure differences between atmospheric air and air in the lungs. To understand how, consider Boyle's law, a principle that describes how gases behave. This law states that the pressure of a gas relates inversely to its volume (provided temperature remains constant). When lung volume increases, intrapulmonic pressure (pressure inside the lungs) drops. When lung volume decreases, intrapulmonic pressure rises.

At each stage of the breathing cycle, pressure gradient shifts regulate air movement. As one expiration ends, before the next inspiration begins, intrapulmonic pressure equals atmospheric pressure (about 760 mm Hg). No air enters or leaves the lungs under these conditions. During inspiration, the chest expands, lung volume increases, and intrapulmonic pressure drops about 1 mm Hg, establishing a pressure gradient. Obeying the gradient, air moves from the atmosphere into the respiratory tract. During expiration, chest capacity decreases, lung volume decreases, and intrapulmonic pressure increases to about 761 mm Hg. Air now travels out of the lungs into the atmosphere, until the pressures are again equalized.

The mechanism of inspiration

As respiratory muscles contract, the thorax enlarges and lung volume increases, establishing a pressure gradient that draws atmospheric air into the lungs.

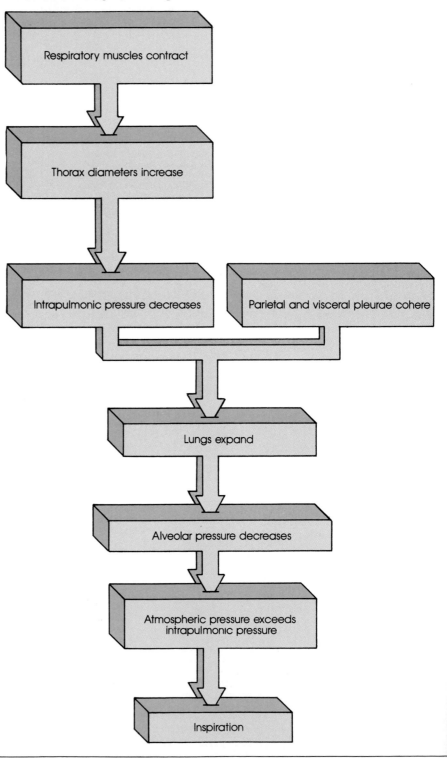

The mechanism of expiration
The respiratory muscles relax, decreasing thorax size and increasing intrapulmonic pressure. The new pressure gradient forces air out through the respiratory tract.

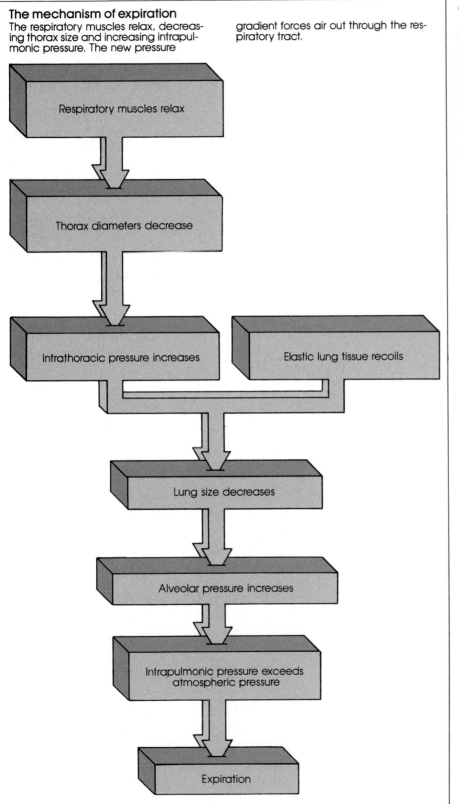

Respiratory muscles relax

Thorax diameters decrease

Intrathoracic pressure increases

Elastic lung tissue recoils

Lung size decreases

Alveolar pressure increases

Intrapulmonic pressure exceeds atmospheric pressure

Expiration

THE WORK OF BREATHING
A healthy person uses just 2% to 3% of his body's total energy for normal quiet breathing. But a patient with a pulmonary disorder may spend a third or more of his energy on respiration.

The work of breathing is determined by four factors: lung elastance, lung compliance, airway resistance, and, of course, the volume of air breathed. When one or more of these physical forces increases or decreases, breathing becomes more laborious. A patient with a severe respiratory disease may die, just from the effort of breathing.

Lung elastance. Because lung tissue is elastic, it has a natural tendency to contract, or recoil, during expiration. This elasticity is due mainly to surface tension, the force that makes two fluids cling together stubbornly when they come into contact. Actually, surface tension between alveolar air and fluid in the alveolar lining is so great that it would cause alveolar collapse were it not countered by another factor—surfactant. A lipoprotein mixture secreted by alveolar epithelial cells, surfactant acts as a buffer, preventing contact between alveolar air and fluid and reducing surface tension 2- to 14-fold. Without adequate surfactant, the lungs would collapse. For example, newborn infants with respiratory distress syndrome (hyaline membrane disease) don't secrete enough surfactant to counter surface tension. Unable to expand their lungs, these infants may die soon after birth, overwhelmed by the effort of breathing.

Lung compliance. Although the degree of lung elastance determines how much work is required to contract the lungs during expiration, compliance determines how well the alveoli and

CONTINUED ON PAGE 16

MECHANICS CONTINUED

THE WORK OF BREATHING CONTINUED

lung tissues expand during inspiration. Two factors influence compliance: lung expansibility and chest wall expansibility. Any condition that impedes lung compliance increases the work of breathing. In pulmonary fibrosis, tough fibrous tissue replaces the normally elastic lung tissue, making it harder to expand the lungs.

Airway resistance. The wider and shorter the airway, the more easily air flows through it. If accumulated secretions narrow the bronchial radius by 50%, airway resistance increases 16-fold. Endotracheal tubing extends airway length. If your patient's intubated, keep in mind that, if the tube doubles airway length, resistance becomes twice as strong.

The pattern of airflow through the respiratory passages also affects airway resistance. *Laminar flow*, a linear pattern that occurs at low rates, offers minimal resistance. This flow type occurs mainly in the small peripheral airways of the bronchial tree. The eddying pattern of *turbulent flow* creates friction and increases resistance. Turbulent flow is normal in the trachea and large central bronchi. But if the smaller airways become constricted or clogged with secretions, turbulent flow may occur there also. A mixed pattern known as *transitional flow* is common at lower flow rates in the larger airways, particularly where the airways meet, branch, or narrow from obstruction.

Obesity, late-term pregnancy, ascites, and abdominal distention can also increase the work of breathing by creating nonelastic resistance. The diaphragm and abdominal contents exert a force that inhibits downward thoracic expansion. You can make breathing easier for a patient with one of these conditions by elevating the head of his bed.

LUNG VOLUMES AND CAPACITIES

Broken down into volumes and capacities, the quantities of air exchanged in breathing represent the amounts inspired and expired under various conditions, as well as the amounts that remain in the lungs at certain stages of the breathing cycle.

To ensure proper gas exchange between alveolar air and pulmonary capillary blood, air quantities must be normal. If your patient has a respiratory disorder, the doctor will order pulmonary function studies to measure volumes and capacities. (To find out how to interpret pulmonary function tests, read page 38.)

Body build, gender, age, and athletic conditioning can affect air quantities. Pulmonary volumes and capacities may decrease with age. They're about 25% higher in men than in women, and higher in a large, athletic person than in one who's small and thin.

Most measurements of volume and capacity are also higher if taken while the patient's standing erect. When he's lying or sitting, inspiration's restricted by abdominal contents pressing against the diaphragm. And since more blood flows into the lungs when he lies down, there's also less space available for air.

Volumes. The volume of air a person inspires or expires with each normal breath (about 4.5 to 6.0 liters) is known as tidal volume (V_T). But a person can force additional air into or out of his lungs in the same way he'd blow up a balloon. Forcibly inhaling, he can draw in an extra 3 liters. This amount is referred to as inspiratory reserve volume (IRV). Its counterpart, expiratory reserve volume (ERV), represents the volume of air he can expire after normal expiration. ERV's usually about 1.1 liters.

Airflow patterns

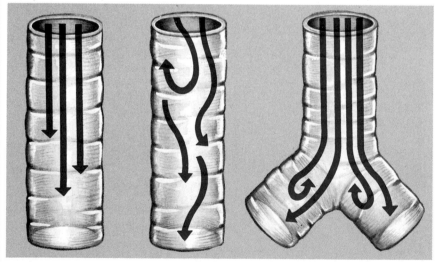

Laminar flow
This linear pattern, found mostly in the small peripheral bronchial passages, offers minimal resistance.

Turbulent flow
Normal in the trachea and large central bronchi, where flow rates are high, this eddying pattern increases resistance.

Transitional flow
In low-flow regions—for example, where larger airways join or branch—this mixed pattern occurs.

Air volumes exchanged in ventilation

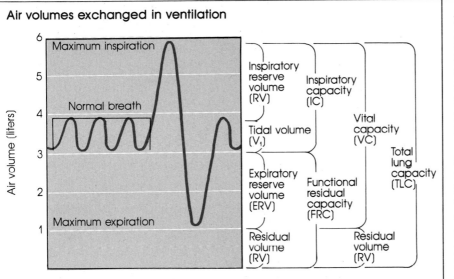

The spirogram (plotted in blue) shows a patient's tidal volume and maximum inspiration and expiration capabilities.

Other vital pulmonary functions can be calculated from these values, as shown above.

But no matter how hard a person tries, he can't force all the air out of his lungs. About 1.2 liters remain trapped in the alveoli. This residual air, called residual volume (RV), performs an important function: it aerates the blood between breaths. Without RV, oxygen and carbon dioxide levels in the blood would fluctuate widely with each respiration. Air remains in the lungs even after death. Minimal volume, the air trapped inside the alveoli by bronchiolar collapse, is sufficient to make a lung removed from the body float on water.

You can determine your patient's minute respiratory volume (V_E) if you know his V_T and respiratory rate. Just multiply the two amounts. If V_T is 0.45 liters and the respiratory rate's 12 breaths per minute, V_E is about 5.4 liters.

Capacities. Lung capacities are combinations of two or more volumes. Vital capacity (VC), the largest volume of air a person can move in and out of his lungs, is determined by having the patient expire with maximum force after the deepest possible inhalation. Thus, VC equals V_T + ERV + IRV. The average young man's VC is about 4.6 liters; the average woman's, about 3.1 liters.

Inspiratory capacity (IC) is the maximum amount of air a person can inhale after normal expiration. To determine IC, add V_T and IRV. Average IC is about 3.5 liters.

The amount of air remaining in the lungs after normal expiration determines functional residual capacity (FRC). Normally about 2.3 liters, FRC's higher in a patient with chronic obstructive pulmonary disease (COPD), from increased amounts of air trapped in the alveoli. It's lower in a patient with adult respiratory distress syndrome (ARDS) or hyaline membrane disease, because alveolar collapse makes the lungs stiff and hard to expand.

The maximum amount of air the lungs and respiratory passages can hold after the most forceful inspiration is the total lung capacity (TLC). TLC's equal to the sum of all four lung volumes (V_T + IRV + ERV + RV). Average TLC's roughly 5.8 liters.

ALVEOLAR VENTILATION: THE CRUCIAL MEASURE

Perhaps the most important measure of pulmonary function is alveolar ventilation (V_A)—the volume of air that actually reaches the alveoli. Only this air takes part in the gas exchange with blood.

Alveolar ventilation constitutes about two thirds of the tidal volume—the air inspired in a normal breath. The remaining air fills the upper airways (nose, pharynx, larynx, trachea, bronchi, and bronchioles). Because these passages aren't perfused by pulmonary capillary blood, no gas exchange occurs here. These regions are thus referred to as anatomic dead space; the air they contain is known as dead space air (V_D). Normally, dead space air is about 0.15 liters.

If your patient has a respiratory disorder that impairs alveolar function (for example, emphysema), he has both physiologic and anatomic dead space. Although many alveoli are ventilated, their blood supply's limited. His physiologic dead space may be as much as 10 times greater than his anatomic dead space (in a healthy person, the two are roughly equal).

Is your patient's alveolar ventilation normal? You can determine this by checking his arterial blood gas measurements. If the carbon dioxide level's elevated, alveolar ventilation's reduced, causing respiratory acidosis. If the carbon dioxide level's decreased, alveolar ventilation's excessive, causing respiratory alkalosis.

GAS EXCHANGE

RESPIRATORY MEMBRANE: WHERE ALVEOLUS AND PULMONARY CAPILLARY MEET

In just one quarter of a second, pulmonary blood swaps oxygen for carbon dioxide through the process of diffusion.

Both gases complete a circuit that takes them from the lungs to tissue cells and back. Drawn into the body with each breath, oxygen enters some 300 million alveoli, awaiting transport to cells, where it's needed for metabolism. Carbon dioxide, a metabolic waste product, takes the opposite route, traveling from the cells to the lungs through pulmonary capillaries. From there it's expired out of the body.

The site of this speedy gas exchange is the respiratory membrane, where the alveolus and pulmonary capillary meet.

The membrane's thinness is the key to rapid diffusion. Although consisting of several alveolar and capillary layers in addition to a fluid lining, the membrane's only 0.004 mm thick. Yet its total surface area is 50 to 100 m²—roughly equivalent to the area of a tennis court. At any given moment, the pulmonary capillaries hold just 60 to 140 ml of blood. Such a small amount spread so thinly permits each corpuscle to get as close as possible to alveolar air, facilitating rapid diffusion.

Any disorder that thickens the respiratory membrane can impair diffusion. In a patient with pulmonary edema, for instance, fluid collects in the interstitial spaces of the membrane and alveoli. Gases must cross both the membrane and surplus fluid, slowing diffusion. Fibrotic lung diseases can have the same effect.

If the membrane thickens to more than two or three times it normal width, gas exchange is seriously impeded.

A patient who's had a lung removed also has a gas transfer deficiency, since the surface area of his respiratory membrane's reduced. So does the emphysema patient, whose membrane surface area is decreased by alveolar destruction. If enough surface area's lost, gas exchange is impaired significantly even when he's resting.

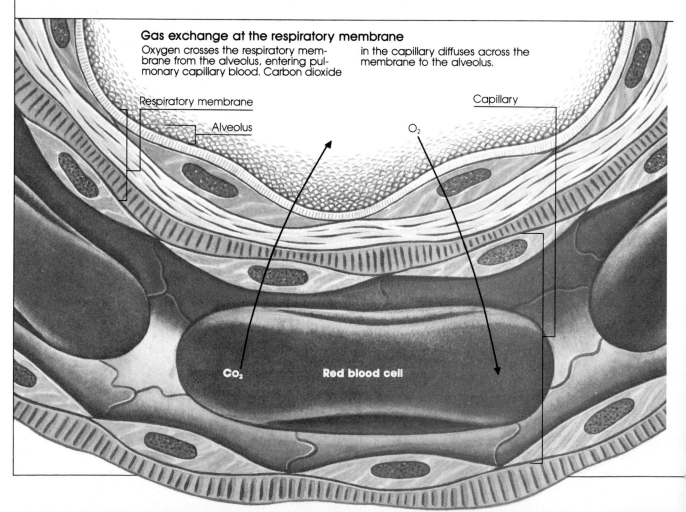

Gas exchange at the respiratory membrane

Oxygen crosses the respiratory membrane from the alveolus, entering pulmonary capillary blood. Carbon dioxide in the capillary diffuses across the membrane to the alveolus.

Respiratory membrane

Alveolus

Capillary

O_2

CO_2

Red blood cell

HOW PRESSURE GRADIENTS GOVERN DIFFUSION

The air we breathe contains oxygen, nitrogen, and trace amounts of carbon dioxide and other gases. Like any gaseous mixture, atmospheric air is pressurized from the constant collision of its molecules. At sea level, the combined force of these collisions exerts a pressure of 760 mm Hg.

But each gas within a mixture also exerts its own pressure independently of the other gases. The pressure of an individual gas is known as its partial pressure (designated by a capital P). Combined, the partial pressures of all gases in a mixture must equal the total pressure of the gas mixture—a phenomenon known as Dalton's law. So the sum of the partial pressures of atmospheric gases is 760 mm Hg at sea level.

You can determine the partial pressure of any gas if you know its concentration in the total mixture. For example, oxygen constitutes 21% of atmospheric air, so its partial pressure is 159 mm Hg (21% of 760). Nitrogen, which makes up 79% of atmospheric air, exerts a partial pressure of 600 mm Hg (79% of 760).

Why are partial pressures important? Because diffusion's achieved through differences in the partial pressures of oxygen and carbon dioxide. Gases diffuse across the respiratory membrane by the same mechanism that causes air to move into and out of the lungs: pressure gradients. As we explained on page 14, a gas moves from a high-pressure area to a low-pressure area until pressures are equalized. In the lungs, where the partial pressure of oxygen is relatively high, oxygen moves down its pressure gradient, diffusing out of the alveoli and across the respiratory membrane into oxygen-poor capillary blood. Carbon dioxide follows its own pressure gradient along the reverse route, passing out of capillary blood, crossing the respiratory membrane, and entering the alveoli. (Nitrogen, an inert gas, doesn't participate in alveolar gas exchange.) Alveolar air has a nearly constant content of 14% to 15% oxygen and 5.5% carbon dioxide.

Anything that decreases the partial pressure of oxygen in the alveoli reduces the pressure gradient between alveolar and capillary oxygen. The result: Less oxygen enters the blood. High altitude has this effect. As atmospheric pressure drops, so does the partial pressure of each atmospheric gas. Less oxygen enters the lungs, the partial pressure of alveolar oxygen decreases, and less oxygen's available for diffusion.

A patient with hypoventilation (reduced ventilation) may also have impaired blood oxygenation. That's why it's important to closely monitor your patient's respiratory rate and depth if he's receiving a drug, such as morphine, that slows respiration. Blood oxygenation also suffers when increased amounts of carbon dioxide displace oxygen in the alveoli.

Physical exercise has a beneficial effect on blood oxygenation, increasing the volume of blood that flows through the lung capillaries while raising the respiration rate.

Pressure gradients and gas exchange

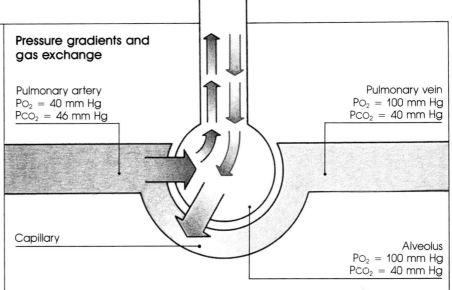

Pulmonary artery
$PO_2 = 40$ mm Hg
$PCO_2 = 46$ mm Hg

Pulmonary vein
$PO_2 = 100$ mm Hg
$PCO_2 = 40$ mm Hg

Capillary

Alveolus
$PO_2 = 100$ mm Hg
$PCO_2 = 40$ mm Hg

Pressure gradients control gas exchange between the alveolus and the pulmonary capillary. High alveolar oxygen pressure forces oxygen (blue arrows) out of the alveolus into the capillary. High capillary carbon dioxide pressure forces carbon dioxide (gray arrows) from the capillary into the alveolus.

Altitude and oxygen pressure

As shown below, the partial pressure of oxygen drops as altitude increases.

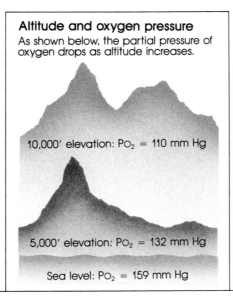

10,000' elevation: $PO_2 = 110$ mm Hg

5,000' elevation: $PO_2 = 132$ mm Hg

Sea level: $PO_2 = 159$ mm Hg

GAS EXCHANGE CONTINUED

MATCHING VENTILATION TO BLOOD FLOW

Effective gas exchange depends on two things: an adequate volume of oxygen reaching the alveoli and sufficient blood flow (perfusion) through pulmonary capillaries.

Actually, it's the relationship between the two that's important. This relationship's described as the ratio of ventilation to perfusion: V/Q.

In the normal lung, ventilation averages 4 liters/minute; perfusion averages 5 liters/minute. So the V/Q ratio's normally 4:5, or 0.8 (4 ÷ 5).

Ideally, ventilation and perfusion would be equally matched and uniformly distributed throughout the lung, producing a V/Q ratio of 1. But this isn't the case, even in the normal, healthy lung. When a person stands erect, the effects of gravity significantly reduce both perfusion and ventilation in his upper lung. But perfusion's affected more than ventilation. The V/Q ratio may be as high as 2.4. The situation's reversed in the lower lung, with perfusion slightly exceeding ventilation.

Inadequate ventilation. When perfusion's normal but ventilation's inadequate, the V/Q ratio's low (less than 0.8). Although blood flows through the pulmonary capillaries, some alveoli aren't being ventilated. Consequently, no gas exchange occurs in the affected lung regions. This pattern's called a shunt. Blood from a shunted lung region returns to the heart's left atrium unoxygenated.

Pneumonia, pulmonary edema, cystic fibrosis, and chronic bronchitis can all reduce ventilation to affected portions of the lung. But even in the normal lung, a small amount of blood (3% to 5% of the heart's total output) is shunted. This is blood from the bronchial vessels and thebesian cardiac veins that normally passes from the right to left side of the heart without participating in gas exchange. This type of shunt's known as anatomic.

A shunt produced by a lung disorder is called an intrapulmonary shunt; the total amount of shunted blood in a patient with both anatomic and intrapulmonary shunts constitutes what's referred to as the physiologic shunt.

Compensating for a low V/Q ratio. The body tries to compensate for an intrapulmonary shunt in several ways. The first is neurochemical. Poor ventilation decreases arterial blood's oxygen level while increasing its carbon dioxide level. Responding to this

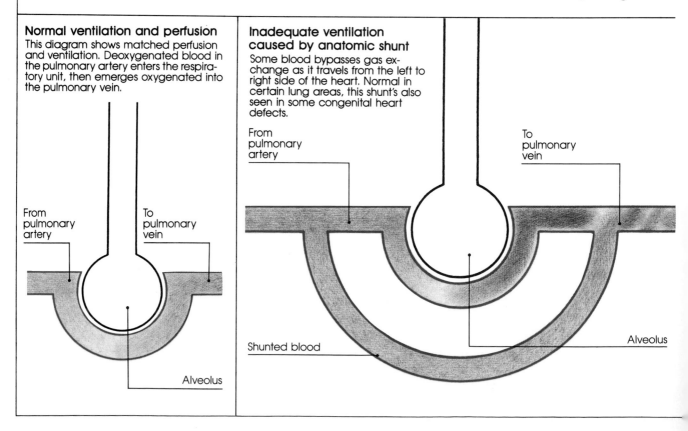

Normal ventilation and perfusion
This diagram shows matched perfusion and ventilation. Deoxygenated blood in the pulmonary artery enters the respiratory unit, then emerges oxygenated into the pulmonary vein.

From pulmonary artery

To pulmonary vein

Alveolus

Inadequate ventilation caused by anatomic shunt
Some blood bypasses gas exchange as it travels from the left to right side of the heart. Normal in certain lung areas, this shunt's also seen in some congenital heart defects.

From pulmonary artery

To pulmonary vein

Shunted blood

Alveolus

change, central chemoreceptors in the brain and peripheral receptors in the carotid and aortic bodies send impulses to the brain's respiratory center. The brain speeds signals to the intercostal and phrenic nerves to increase the rate and depth of breathing, which in turn increases ventilation.

If your patient has advanced lung disease or respiratory failure, this measure alone won't help. A second compensatory mechanism—an increase in *cardiac output*—is usually more efficient. How does this help? To boost cardiac output, the heart rate increases. Blood flows through the capillaries faster, so tissues extract less oxygen from blood.

The body's third response to a low V/Q ratio is localized. Through a mechanism not fully understood, arterioles serving poorly ventilated or collapsed alveoli constrict, diverting blood flow to better-ventilated areas. This creates silent units that have inadequate ventilation and perfusion. These units don't contribute as much to uneven V/Q ratios.

Inadequate perfusion. What happens when a patient's ventilation is normal but his pulmonary blood flow is poor? Again, no gas exchange occurs in the affected lung areas since no blood's available to carry gases away from the alveoli. In this case, the V/Q ratio's higher than normal. Because ventilation to these lung portions is wasted, a high V/Q ratio produces physiologic dead space. (You read about this on page 17.) Hemorrhage, emphysema, and pulmonary embolism can lead to high V/Q ratios.

Compensating for a high V/Q ratio. When many alveoli receive adequate ventilation but poor perfusion, the partial pressure of arterial oxygen decreases, resulting in hypoxemia. The patient becomes short of breath, which causes his respiratory rate and depth to increase and his arterial carbon dioxide level to decrease.

The body's second reaction is to create silent units, probably by stimulating airway resistance in the passages serving the affected capillaries.

Assessing V/Q imbalances. Pulmonary function studies, radiography, and blood gas analysis can determine whether pulmonary ventilation and perfusion are adequate. You'll read about these methods in later sections of the book.

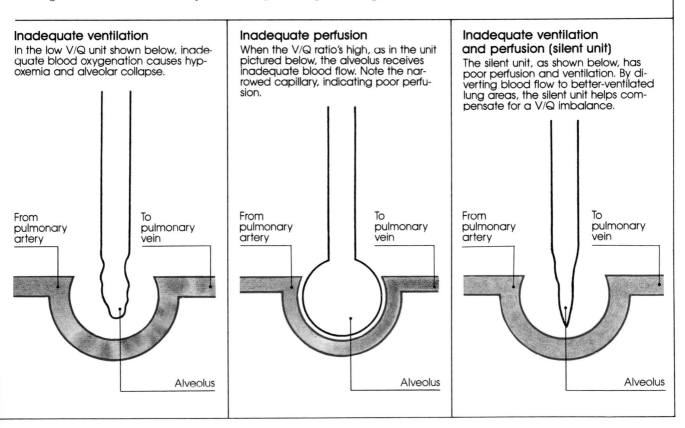

Inadequate ventilation
In the low V/Q unit shown below, inadequate blood oxygenation causes hypoxemia and alveolar collapse.

From pulmonary artery

To pulmonary vein

Alveolus

Inadequate perfusion
When the V/Q ratio's high, as in the unit pictured below, the alveolus receives inadequate blood flow. Note the narrowed capillary, indicating poor perfusion.

From pulmonary artery

To pulmonary vein

Alveolus

Inadequate ventilation and perfusion (silent unit)
The silent unit, as shown below, has poor perfusion and ventilation. By diverting blood flow to better-ventilated lung areas, the silent unit helps compensate for a V/Q imbalance.

From pulmonary artery

To pulmonary vein

Alveolus

GAS EXCHANGE CONTINUED

HOW BLOOD TRANSPORTS GASES

After oxygen diffuses into the bloodstream, it must be transported to body tissues. At the same time, carbon dioxide must be removed from tissues, then carried to the lungs for elimination.

Like any fluid, blood can hold only small amounts of gas in solution. Just 3% of oxygen and 7% of carbon dioxide pass through the bloodstream in a dissolved state. The remaining portions quickly bind with other blood constituents for transport.

About 97% of oxygen combines with hemoglobin, forming oxyhemoglobin. The nature of this chemical union holds the key to oxygen transport: it's reversible. When conditions are appropriate, the union comes undone. Here's how it works: Where oxygen pressure's high (for example, in pulmonary capillaries), oxygen and hemoglobin bind. Where oxygen pressure's low, as it is in tissue capillaries, hemoglobin releases oxygen.

Oxygen capacity. When hemoglobin's completely saturated, each gram can hold about 1.34 ml of oxygen. This amount represents blood's oxygen capacity. Every 100 ml of blood normally contains about 15 g of hemoglobin. So oxygen capacity's normally about 20 ml/100 ml of blood (15×1.34).

Oxyhemoglobin saturation. But the entire oxygen capacity is rarely used. The amount of oxygen actually carried by hemoglobin is called the oxyhemoglobin saturation level. If oxyhemoglobin accounts for 85% of the body's hemoglobin, oxyhemoglobin saturation is 85% in arterial blood.

Oxyhemoglobin saturation determines how much oxygen's delivered to body tissues. Normal body functions require 90% to 100% saturation. A patient with 85% to 89% saturation may be mildly hypoxemic; a saturation level below 84% leads to obvious hypoxemia. When saturation's less than 35%, hypoxemia's usually fatal.

Oxyhemoglobin dissociation curve. Various conditions can alter oxyhemoglobin saturation. But saturation levels depend most on oxygen pressure. The relationship between oxygen pressure and saturation is represented by the oxyhemoglobin dissociation curve (see the graph at left).

The curve's S shape shows that the relationship isn't linear. In other words, a given increase or decrease in oxygen pressure doesn't always result in an equivalent rise or fall in oxyhemoglobin saturation.

The top of the curve depicts conditions in the lung, where oxygen pressure's highest (100 mm Hg) and hemoglobin saturation's nearly total (97.5%). This portion of the curve is flat, revealing that even a fairly large drop in oxygen pressure in the lungs won't reduce saturation significantly.

But, in body tissue cells (represented by the steep part of the curve), saturation decreases substantially with each slight drop in oxygen pressure. Within the cap-

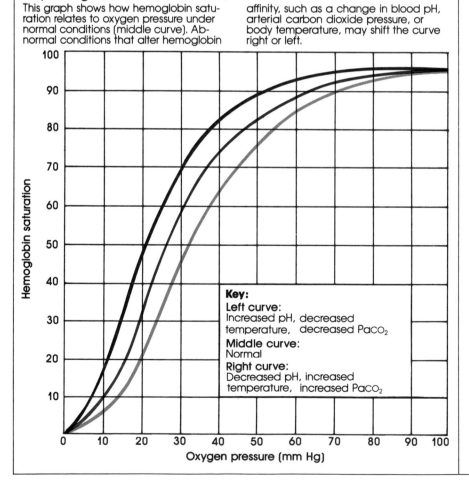

Oxyhemoglobin dissociation curve

This graph shows how hemoglobin saturation relates to oxygen pressure under normal conditions (middle curve). Abnormal conditions that alter hemoglobin affinity, such as a change in blood pH, arterial carbon dioxide pressure, or body temperature, may shift the curve right or left.

Hemoglobin saturation (vertical axis)

Oxygen pressure (mm Hg) (horizontal axis)

Key:
Left curve:
Increased pH, decreased temperature, decreased $PaCO_2$
Middle curve:
Normal
Right curve:
Decreased pH, increased temperature, increased $PaCO_2$

illary, oxygen's easily unloaded from hemoglobin to blood plasma for diffusion into tissue cells.

Shifting the curve. Changes in blood pH, arterial carbon dioxide pressure, and body temperature can alter oxyhemoglobin saturation. As a result, the curve will move to either the left or right on the graph. A drop in pH, a rise in body temperature, or an increase in arterial carbon dioxide pressure will shift the curve to the right. This means that oxyhemoglobin saturation's lower for any given oxygen pressure.

When does the curve shift to the left? When there's a pH elevation, a drop in body temperature, or a reduction in arterial carbon dioxide pressure. As the curve shifts to the left, oxyhemoglobin saturation rises for any given oxygen pressure.

Cardiac output plays an important role in delivering oxygen to body tissues. If a patient's cardiac output (normally 5 liters/minute) drops to half its normal amount, his oxygen delivery also decreases by half. To compensate, body tissues extract as much oxygen from blood as possible. But often, oxygen pressure and capacity are too low to fully compensate for reduced output, so tissue hypoxia results.

Carbon dioxide transport. Because it's highly soluble, carbon dioxide travels easily between the lungs and tissue cells. Even under abnormal conditions, the bloodstream can transport much greater quantities of carbon dioxide than oxygen.

Once carbon dioxide has diffused out of tissue cells into capillaries, a small amount (about 7%) dissolves in plasma. The remainder enters red blood cells, where it forms several types of chemical unions.

About 70% reacts with the

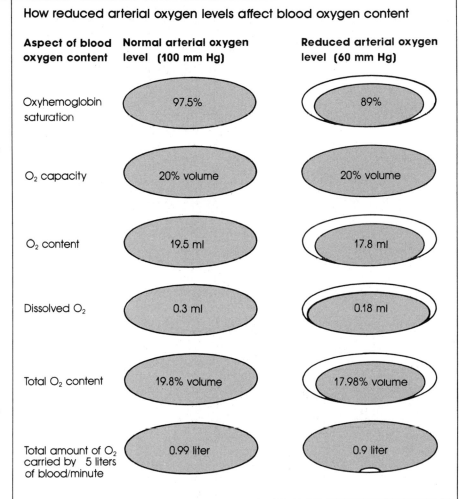

How reduced arterial oxygen levels affect blood oxygen content

Aspect of blood oxygen content	Normal arterial oxygen level (100 mm Hg)	Reduced arterial oxygen level (60 mm Hg)
Oxyhemoglobin saturation	97.5%	89%
O_2 capacity	20% volume	20% volume
O_2 content	19.5 ml	17.8 ml
Dissolved O_2	0.3 ml	0.18 ml
Total O_2 content	19.8% volume	17.98% volume
Total amount of O_2 carried by 5 liters of blood/minute	0.99 liter	0.9 liter

water in blood to form carbonic acid. This reversible combination's the most important means of carbon dioxide transport. Catalyzed by the carbonic anhydrase enzyme, carbonic acid's formed 5,000 times faster than it would be in plasma, where the enzyme's lacking. The reaction reaches almost total equilibrium within a fraction of a second.

Then, almost instantly, carbonic acid dissociates into hydrogen and bicarbonate ions. The ions go their separate ways: hydrogen ions link with hemoglobin, and bicarbonate ions diffuse through the cell membrane into the plasma.

Carbon dioxide also reacts directly with hemoglobin, forming the compound carbaminohemoglobin. About 30% of the carbon dioxide in the body is transported to the lungs in this form.

During carbon dioxide transport, blood becomes more acidic as a result of carbonic acid formation. Under normal conditions, this doesn't create problems since blood contains a buffer that prevents extreme pH changes. But when metabolism's very rapid, as it is during exercise and certain disease states, pH in the tissues may fall as much as 0.5 or more. Acidosis may result.

GAS EXCHANGE CONTINUED

INTERNAL RESPIRATION: THE INSIDE STORY

Internal respiration—gas exchange between tissue cells and systemic capillary blood—in many ways resembles gas exchange in the lungs. But now pressure gradients carry oxygen and carbon dioxide in directions opposite those they traveled across the respiratory membrane.

Carbon dioxide's under higher pressure in tissue cells (where it's produced by catabolism) than it is in systemic blood. Yielding to this pressure gradient, carbon dioxide diffuses out of cells, then combines with hemoglobin in systemic blood to form carbaminohemoglobin.

Oxygen pressure's lower in tissue cells than in systemic blood. Following its pressure gradient, oxygen dissociates gradually from oxyhemoglobin, diffusing into tissue cells one molecule at a time. Blood's never devoid of oxygen. At the end of each circulatory cycle, some oxygen remains in the blood.

Gas exchange in tissue capillaries

Oxyhemoglobin in the tissue capillary releases oxygen (O_2), which then diffuses into the tissue cell (shown in close-up at left). Carbon dioxide (CO_2) diffuses in the opposite direction, entering systemic blood to form carbaminohemoglobin.

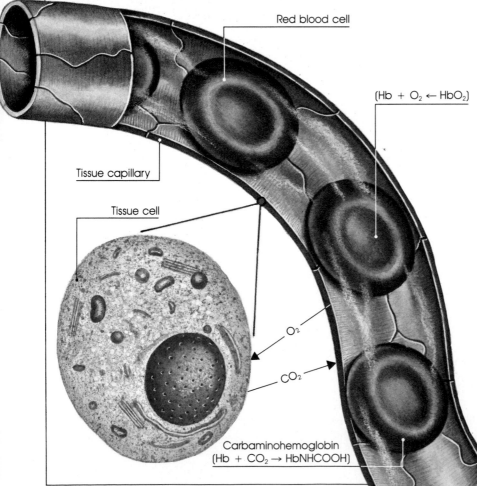

Red blood cell

$(Hb + O_2 \leftarrow HbO_2)$

Tissue capillary

Tissue cell

O_2

CO_2

Carbaminohemoglobin
$(Hb + CO_2 \rightarrow HbNHCOOH)$

WHEN NITROGEN'S A PROBLEM

Four fifths of the air we breathe is nitrogen. At sea level, nitrogen has no known effect on the body. It dissolves in the blood and body tissue.

But when atmospheric pressure's high, nitrogen can create problems. A deep-sea diver may develop decompression sickness (the bends) as increased pressure below sea level causes more nitrogen than usual to dissolve in the bloodstream. After a few hours, body tissues become nitrogen saturated. If the diver rises to the surface too quickly, nitrogen bubbles form inside body fluids and tissue. Bubbles in peripheral nerves or the central nervous system (CNS) can cause symptoms ranging from localized pain, dizziness, and fatigue to permanent paralysis or mental disturbances. If bubbles form in the blood and block lung capillaries, the diver may develop severe dyspnea followed by pulmonary edema.

To prevent decompression sickness, a diver must rise to the surface gradually to allow excess nitrogen to escape from the dissolved state slowly. Safe decompression time depends on both the depth to which he descended and the time he remained there. A diver who worked for an hour at a depth of 190' needs 3 hours to decompress.

Narcosis. Nitrogen can also have the intoxicating effect known as nitrogen narcosis. Like other anesthetic gases, nitrogen dissolves freely in membranes or other lipid structures of nerve cells, reducing the cells' excitability. The diver may experience symptoms of euphoria at 120' and become weak and clumsy as he descends further. Beyond 300', nitrogen narcosis usually incapacitates him.

EMERGENCY ASSESSMENT
PHYSICAL EXAMINATION
DIAGNOSTIC TESTS

EMERGENCY ASSESSMENT

CASE IN POINT

RECOGNIZING A RESPIRATORY CRISIS

Your patient, Joanne Landis, a 32-year-old accountant, is recovering from a cesarean section and is now in a medical/surgical unit because of her uncontrolled diabetes. Since the surgery, 48 hours ago, Mrs. Landis has remained immobile, complaining that she's too tired and in too much pain—despite administration of 50 mg of meperidine (Demerol) every 4 hours—to get up. She's refused incentive spirometry and, despite your urging, has not been coughing or breathing deeply. Also, she's removed her antiembolism stockings.

Suddenly, Mrs. Landis calls for a nurse, and when you enter her room, you find her gasping for air. Quickly assessing the situation, you realize her airway's open and she's alert, indicating adequate oxygen intake. You call another nurse to bring Mrs. Landis' chart and contact her doctor. Then, you ask: "Do you have any chest pain?" She apprehensively answers, "Yes." Next, while taking her vital signs, you ask, "Is the pain severe?" "Yes, it's sharp, like someone is stabbing me," she answers. Her pulse is high—112. Her blood pressure is 128/86; respirations 28; and temperature 101°F. (38.3°C.). You review her chart for her baseline vital signs—pulse 76, blood pressure 110/70, respirations 16, and temperature 98.2° F. (36.8°C.). On auscultation, you hear decreased breath sounds and rales at the anterior base of her right lung.

Considering the circum-stances, you suspect pulmonary embolism. Her history supports your suspicions: Mrs. Landis has smoked two packs of cigarettes a day for 11 years. Also, her family history includes thrombophlebitis.

The doctor orders a chest X-ray, EKG, and an ABG analysis. While her EKG is normal, her chest X-ray reveals a density in the base of the right lung that wasn't there preoperatively. Furthermore, ABG measurements reveal low PaO_2 (73), indicating hypoxia; low $PaCO_2$ (33), indicating hypocapnia from hyperventilation; and a slightly alkaline serum pH level (7.47). While a lung scan is needed to confirm a diagnosis, all indicators point to pulmonary embolism.

Your role. How do *you* respond when your patient suddenly develops a respiratory emergency? While the situation's urgency forces you to juggle several assessment steps simultaneously, you can remain calm and complete a thorough assessment in minutes by taking the following important steps:
• Assess ABCs (airway, breathing, and circulation) immediately. For details, see the next page.
• Administer oxygen. However, before you do, consider the patient's *primary* condition. For example, suppose your steroid-dependent asthmatic patient has an acute attack and is in respiratory crisis. He needs corticosteroids to control his bronchial inflammation before you can administer oxygen.

Furthermore, the patient with chronic obstructive pulmonary disease (COPD) needs a slight oxygen deficiency to stimulate his breathing. Although he needs oxygen during a crisis, administering high concentrations will increase his arterial oxygen level so much that he'll stop breathing. Remember, patients with COPD take a breath because their arterial oxygen level gets too low. Instead, administer 2 liters/minute, or as ordered.
• Call for help. Ask another nurse to bring the patient's chart and contact his doctor. Don't leave the patient alone until his breathing is stable.
• Ask the patient only questions to which he can answer yes or no—to save his breath and your time. Specifically question him about key symptoms, such as chest pain or cough. His reply may reveal changes in his voice, indicating upper airway obstruction. Also, his reply will help you again assess his mental status.
• Take his vital signs and compare them with the baseline vital signs recorded on his chart.
• Perform a brief physical examination, again consulting his chart for baseline information.
• Arrange laboratory tests, as ordered.

THE ABCs OF A RESPIRATORY EMERGENCY

Your first priority in a respiratory emergency is always to assess your patient's ABCs—airway, breathing, and circulation. Use this chart as a guide in performing a thorough 90-second emergency assessment to determine your patient's condition and establish your nursing care priorities.

A is for airway
Goal: Establish an open airway
Nursing interventions:
• Check your patient's airway for signs of obstruction: wheezing, stridor, or choking.
• If you suspect an airway obstruction, position your patient on his back with his neck hyperextended. (If he makes a violent effort to sit up, let him. This may be a reflex action to establish an open airway.) Open his mouth by pulling down his lower lip as shown in the top photo. Then sweep two fingers deep into his mouth to remove any foreign matter (see bottom photo).

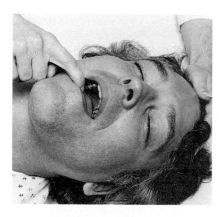

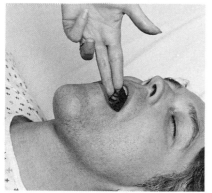

B is for breathing
Goal: Restore adequate respirations
Nursing interventions:
• Check your patient's breathing to determine if his respirations are adequate. Look, listen, and feel for signs of breathing (see top photo).
• Observe the quality of your patient's respirations.
• If your patient has stopped breathing, begin giving rescue breaths (see bottom photo).
• If your patient's breathing is distressed, auscultate breath sounds bilaterally. Document your findings in his chart.

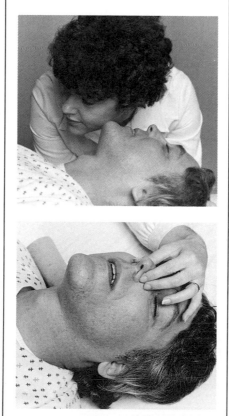

C is for circulation
Goal: Maintain adequate perfusion
Nursing interventions:
• Check your patient's circulation by feeling for a pulse in the carotid artery. As shown in the top photo, check the carotid pulse on the side closest to you. If he has a neck injury, feel instead for a femoral pulse.
• If no pulse exists, begin CPR immediately. (See the bottom photo for proper hand placement during chest compressions.) Brain damage or death occurs if circulation isn't restored in 4 to 6 minutes after respiratory arrest.

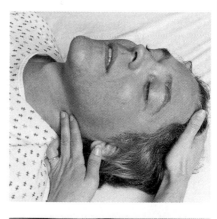

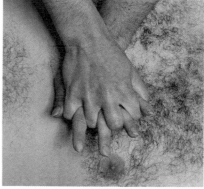

EMERGENCY ASSESSMENT

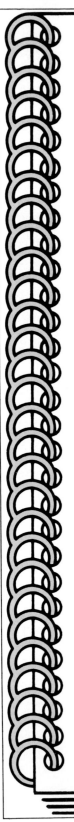

CRITICAL QUESTIONS

EVALUATING YOUR PATIENT'S SIGNS AND SYMPTOMS

As you assess your patient, ask him about his respiratory signs and symptoms. In most cases, these include dyspnea, chest pain, or coughing. In an emergency, you may have to rely on your own observations and the information on the patient's chart. But, if time and the patient's condition allow, question him using this checklist as a guide.

Dyspnea
• When did you first become short of breath?
• Do you have frequent attacks of breathlessness?
• Does body position or time of day affect your breathing?
• Does a particular activity make you feel short of breath?
• What relieves your attacks? What makes them worse?
• Do your lips and nail beds turn blue during an attack?
• Do you have any other signs and symptoms, such as coughing, sweating, or chest pain?
• Has your breathlessness stayed about the same, or is it getting worse?
• Is it combined with wheezing or crowing sounds?

Chest pain
• When did you first notice the chest pain?
• Is it constant, or does it come and go?
• Does the pain stay in one place, or does it spread?
• Does a specific activity cause pain?
• Is the pain accompanied by other signs and symptoms, such as coughing or shortness of breath?
• Does the pain occur when you breathe deeply? Does splinting relieve the pain?
• Have you ever had a chest injury?

Cough
• How long have you had the cough? Does anything make it worse?
• Does the cough occur at a specific time of day?
• Have you recently been exposed to anyone with a similar cough?
• Are you coughing up sputum? If so, does the sputum contain mucus or look frothy? What color is it? Does it have an odor?
• Are you taking any medications for the cough?
• Do you smoke?
• Do you have any allergies?

REVIEWING YOUR PATIENT'S HISTORY

When you review your patient's chart, consider his medical, family, and social history as part of your overall patient assessment. Use the following questions as a guide.

Medical history. Has the patient had any previous respiratory illness (such as pneumonia or asthma), heart disease or invasive procedure (such as bronchoscopy or thoracentesis), chest injury or chest surgery (such as thoracoplasty or pneumonectomy)? How often does he get colds?

Does he have any allergies to animals, foods, dust, pollen, or medications? If so, what type of allergic reaction does he have—coughing, sneezing, dyspnea? Has he ever been treated for the allergy?

Also, note any medications the patient's currently taking. His symptom could be the result of a drug interaction or adverse reaction. Is he complying with his medication regimen? Has the patient ever been vaccinated for pneumonia or flu?

Family history. Does anyone in the patient's family have:
• asthma
• emphysema
• chronic allergies
• repeated respiratory problems, such as frequent colds or flu
• cardiovascular problems, such as hypertension or myocardial infarction
• thrombophlebitis
• obesity
• neuromuscular dysfunction?

Social history. Does the patient smoke? How long has he smoked? How much does he smoke, expressed in pack years (the number of cigarette packs smoked per day times the number of years the patient's smoked)?

PHYSICAL EXAMINATION

ASSESSING ENVIRONMENTAL INFLUENCES

The following occupations may predispose your patient to a respiratory disorder:

HIGH-RISK OCCUPATION

Mining (lead, coal, copper, silver, and gold); foundry and pottery work; sandstone and granite cutting
Possible disorder
Silicosis

HIGH-RISK OCCUPATION

Coal mining
Possible disorder
Coal worker's pneumoconiosis (black lung disease) from long-term exposure to coal dust along with excessive cigarette smoking

HIGH-RISK OCCUPATION

Work in chemical, military, ceramic, and aerospace industries; contact with beryllium
Possible disorder
Berylliosis (beryllium disease, Wegener's granulomatosis) from exposure to dust or fumes containing beryllium or its compounds

HIGH-RISK OCCUPATION

Work involving the mining, milling, manufacturing, or application of asbestos products, such as brake lining or insulation
Possible disorder
Asbestosis

HIGH-RISK OCCUPATION

Work in cotton, leather, beer, wood, detergent, flax, and hemp industries
Possible disorder
Asthma from exposure to irritants or allergenic particles or vapors

MODIFYING THE PHYSICAL EXAMINATION

In a respiratory crisis, you may not have time to perform a thorough physical examination. On the next few pages, we'll explain which assessment procedures will provide the best information in an emergency and how to tailor an examination to your patient's condition.

Under routine circumstances, you'd inspect, palpate, percuss, and auscultate—in that order. However, in most respiratory emergencies, you should inspect and auscultate first, since these techniques provide more valuable information about your patient's disorder. Of course, if time allows or if you suspect your patient has a condition that palpation or percussion would reveal, perform these assessment procedures immediately. For example, if you suspect pleural effusion or pneumothorax, percuss first to instantly confirm or rule out your suspicion.

Ongoing assessment. Even before you start physically examining your patient, observe his signs and symptoms. For example, while evaluating his airway, breathing, and circulation and taking his history and vital signs, note his general appearance. Is he having difficulty breathing? Does he seem alert?

Also watch for these clues:
• **Use of accessory muscles.** Is he leaning forward, pulling on the supraclavicular, sternocleidomastoid, intercostal, or abdominal wall muscles? He's probably developed dyspnea.
• **Changed mental status.** Anxiety or agitation suggests decreased oxygenation—hypoxia. Confusion may indicate more severe hypoxia.
• **Cyanosis or finger clubbing.** While both are signs of hypoxia, cyanosis indicates *severe* hypoxia.

• **Chest deformity.** This suggests a preexisting respiratory problem that may have been recently aggravated. (See the next page.)
• **Abnormal respiratory pattern.** (See the next page.)

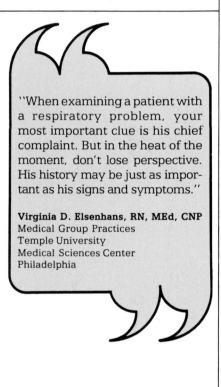

"When examining a patient with a respiratory problem, your most important clue is his chief complaint. But in the heat of the moment, don't lose perspective. His history may be just as important as his signs and symptoms."

Virginia D. Elsenhans, RN, MEd, CNP
Medical Group Practices
Temple University
Medical Sciences Center
Philadelphia

PHYSICAL EXAMINATION CONTINUED

IDENTIFYING CHEST DEFORMITIES

Use this guide to review the physical characteristics, signs, and conditions associated with the three common chest deformities we've illustrated below.

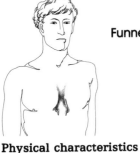

Funnel chest

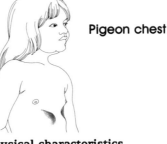

Pigeon chest

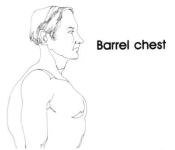

Barrel chest

Physical characteristics
Sinking or funnel-shaped depression of lower sternum; diminished anteroposterior chest diameter
Signs and associated conditions
Postural disorders, such as forward displacement of neck and shoulders; upper thoracic kyphosis; protuberant abdomen; functional heart murmur

Physical characteristics
Projection of sternum beyond abdomen's frontal plane. Evident in two variations: projection greatest at xiphoid process; projection greatest at or near center of sternum
Signs and associated conditions
Functional cardiovascular or respiratory disorders

Physical characteristics
Enlarged anteroposterior and transverse chest dimensions; chest appears barrel-shaped; prominent accessory muscles
Signs and associated conditions
Chronic respiratory disorders; increasing shortness of breath; chronic cough; wheezing

ASSESSING RESPIRATORY PATTERNS

For the most accurate assessment of your patient's respiratory rate, rhythm, and depth, examine him when he's not aware that you're counting his respirations. Otherwise, he may alter his natural breathing pattern.

Count respirations for at least one minute. If you count for less than a minute and then multiply, your count may be off by as many as four respirations per minute. Your patient's respiratory pattern should be even, except for an occasional deep breath.

Use this chart to help you make an accurate assessment.

Eupnea

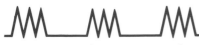

Normal respiratory rate and depth, regular rhythm. Expiration lasts twice as long as inspiration. Adult rate is 16 to 18 breaths per minute.

Tachypnea

Increased respiratory rate, shallow depth; regular or irregular rhythm. Respiration rate also increases with pain or anxiety.

Bradypnea

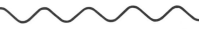

Decreased respiratory rate, variable depth, regular rhythm. Normal during sleep. Abnormal when the brain's respiratory control center is affected by respiratory decompensation.

Biot's

Increased respiratory rate and depth, with irregular periods of apnea between respirations; each breath has the same depth. Usually seen with central nervous system (CNS) disorders.

Cheyne-Stokes

Gradually increasing, then decreasing rate and depth in a cycle lasting 30 to 170 seconds. Alternates with 20- to 60-second periods of apnea; occurs in increased ICP, severe CHF, renal failure, meningitis, and drug overdose.

Kussmaul's

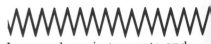

Increased respiratory rate and depth, irregular rhythm. Patient's breathing usually sounds labored; breaths resemble sighs. Also called air hunger or paroxysmal dyspnea. Occurs in renal failure or metabolic acidosis.

AUSCULTATING FOR BREATH SOUNDS

After inspection, lung auscultation is your best assessment tool for most respiratory emergencies. It can detect a bronchial obstruction or air or fluid in the pleural space.

To auscultate, listen with a stethoscope over all lung fields anteriorly, posteriorly, and laterally, if time allows. Follow the sequence shown at right.

Press the stethoscope diaphragm firmly against the patient's skin, wetting his chest hairs if possible to reduce rubbing sounds. Have the patient inhale and exhale slowly and deeply through his mouth.

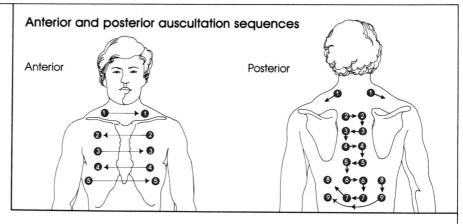

Anterior and posterior auscultation sequences

Anterior   Posterior

Compare the sounds on each side of his chest to distinguish normal from adventitious sounds. (See the chart below and *Identifying adventitious sounds* on the following page.)

Note: If your patient is lying on his side, his uppermost lung will be better ventilated. Keep this in mind when comparing breath sounds.

NURSE'S GUIDE TO NORMAL BREATH SOUNDS

NORMAL BREATH SOUND	DESCRIPTION	POSITION IN RESPIRATORY CYCLE	TYPICAL RESPIRATORY CYCLE	NORMAL FINDINGS	ABNORMAL FINDINGS
Vesicular	• High-pitched and loud on inspiration; low-pitched and soft on expiration	• More prominent during inspiration than during expiration	• Inspiration is longer than expiration, with no pause between them.	• Over peripheral lung fields, you'll hear sounds with a soft, swishy quality.	• Decreased sounds over peripheral lung fields; may indicate emphysema or early pneumonia
Bronchial or tracheal	• High-pitched, loud, harsh, hollow	• Less prominent during inspiration than during expiration	• Inspiration is shorter than expiration, with a pause between them.	• Over the trachea or the mainstem bronchus, you'll hear a sound like air blowing through a hollow tube.	• Bronchial sounds over peripheral lung fields; may indicate atelectasis or consolidation
Bronchovesicular	• Medium to high-pitched, muffled	• Equally prominent during inspiration and expiration	• Inspiration and expiration are equal, with no pause between them.	• Over large airways, either side of the sternum, the angle of Louis, and between the scapulae, you'll hear a blowing sound.	• Bronchovesicular sounds over peripheral lung fields; may indicate consolidation

PHYSICAL EXAMINATION CONTINUED

IDENTIFYING ADVENTITIOUS SOUNDS

Adventitious breath sounds occur when air passes through narrowed airways or moisture, or when the membranes lining the lungs and chest cavity become inflamed. During auscultation, you may hear adventitious sounds superimposed over your patient's normal breath sounds.

Study the chart below to review the features and significance of adventitious sounds. *Note:* Absent breath sounds are also significant and indicate loss of ventilating power. Absent sounds may signify:
• an obstruction of the larynx, trachea, or bronchus
• laryngeal bronchospasm
• pneumonectomy or phrenic nerve palsy
• a malpositioned endotracheal tube
• pleural abnormalities.

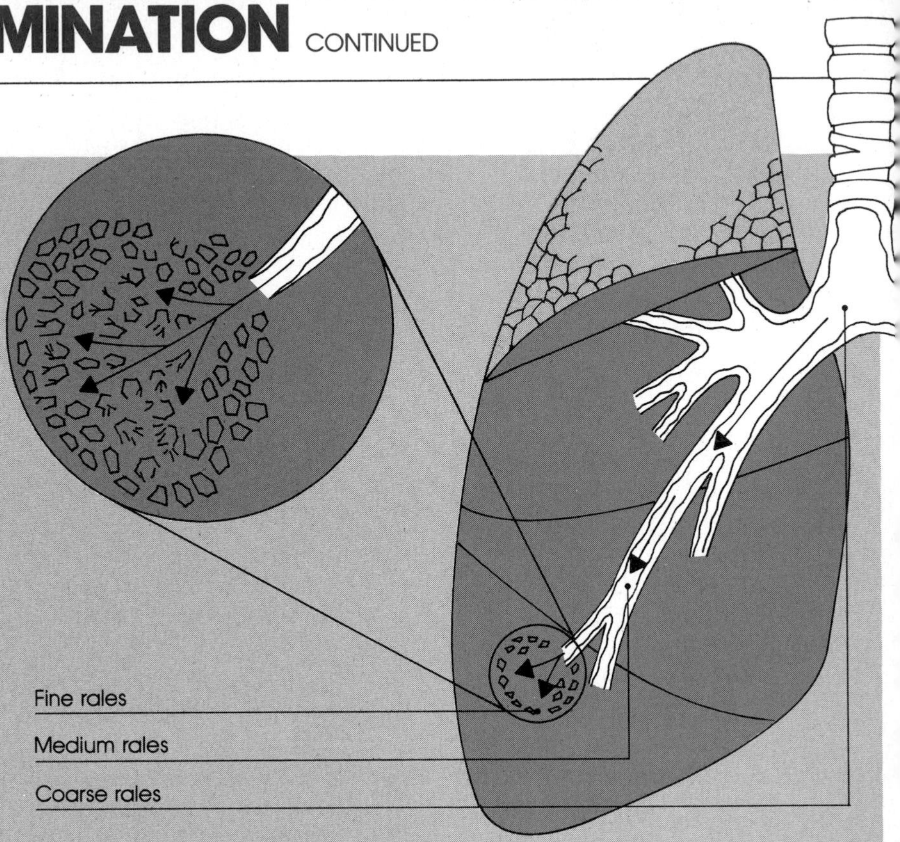

Fine rales

Medium rales

Coarse rales

FINE RALES (CREPITANT)	MEDIUM RALES	RHONCHI (COARSE RALES)	WHEEZING	PLEURAL FRICTION RUB
Description High-pitched, soft crackling and popping	**Description** Medium-pitched bubbling, gurgling, and rattling	**Description** Low-pitched, loud, often musical rattling, bubbling, or gurgling	**Description** High-pitched, squeaky whistling	**Description** Low-pitched, coarse grating or crunching
Position in respiratory cycle End of inspiration	**Position in respiratory cycle** Mid-to-late inspiration	**Position in respiratory cycle** Beginning of inspiration	**Position in respiratory cycle** Most common during expiration	**Position in respiratory cycle** Loudest on inspiration (sounds don't clear with coughing)
Possible cause Fluid in or around the alveoli	**Possible cause** Fluid in or around bronchioles	**Possible cause** Fluid in the bronchi and trachea	**Possible cause** Narrowing of airways from swelling or obstruction	**Possible cause** Inflamed surfaces of pleurae rubbing together
Possible problems Pneumonia, congestive heart failure (CHF), or atelectasis	**Possible problems** CHF, pneumonia, pulmonary edema, bronchitis, bronchiectasis, or lung abscess	**Possible problems** Pneumonia, asthma, emphysema, severe pulmonary edema, or severe bronchitis	**Possible problems** Asthma, emphysema, bronchospasm, foreign body obstruction, mucus obstruction, stenosis, or pulmonary edema	**Possible problems** Pleurisy, tuberculosis, pulmonary infarction, pneumonia, or pulmonary embolism

CHEST PALPATION

During a routine examination, you'd palpate your patient's anterior and posterior chest. However, in a respiratory emergency, palpate only the anterior chest.

Begin by checking for tenderness, broken bones, or wounds. (A hospitalized patient may have undiagnosed broken bones from an unreported accident in his room, such as falling out of bed.) Next check for symmetrical chest expansion. Place your palms on either side of the patient's upper chest, rest your fingers on his shoulders, and extend your thumbs until they meet. Ask the patient to inhale and exhale deeply. Observe the movement of your thumbs on his chest for unilateral lag, which may indicate pleural thickening, atelectasis, pneumothorax, obstruction of a major bronchus, or a misplaced endotracheal tube.

Next, examine his midchest by placing your hands on the sides of his chest. Rest your thumbs at the sixth rib level, and extend them so they meet, as shown in the illustration below. Again, have the patient inhale and exhale deeply. As he inhales, your thumbs will separate. Repeat the examination on his lower chest.

Tactile fremitus. To assess tactile fremitus, position your palms against either side of your pa-

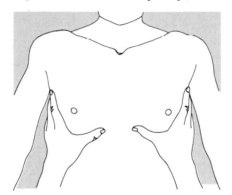

tient's upper chest. Ask him to repeat the words "ninety-nine." As he does, move your palms from his upper to lower chest.

In his upper chest, close to the bronchi, expect to feel fremitus of equal intensity on either side. Greater intensity on one side may signify tissue consolidation. Reduced intensity may indicate emphysema, pneumothorax, or pleural effusion. Anything lying between the vibrations and your hand—for example, air or pleuritic fluid—can decrease or mask fremitus. In the lower chest, you should feel little or no fremitus.

Crepitus. Be alert for any crepitus—crackling noises indicating trapped air within the tissues—especially around wounds, subclavian catheters, and chest tubes.

PERCUSSION: RECOGNIZING CHEST SOUNDS

After palpation, if time allows, percuss your patient's chest anteriorly, posteriorly, and laterally, following the same sequence you used to auscultate (see page 31). Percussion helps to detect a collapsed lung, increased air volume, or fluid in the pleural space.

Anterior percussion. Begin by palpating the supraclavicular areas, comparing right and left sides. Then percuss downward in 2" (5-cm) intervals. Expect to hear the following sounds:
• resonance (a hollow sound) over normal, air-filled lungs
• dullness (a thudding sound) over the diaphragm or over solid or fluid-filled organs, such as the heart and liver. Dullness over the lungs may indicate fluid or solid tissue (consolidation).
• flatness (an extremely dull sound) over the sternum, chest

muscles, or an atelectatic lung
• tympany (a drumlike sound) over the air-filled stomach; tympany over the lungs may mean increased air volume, as in pneumothorax
• hyperresonance (a booming sound) over hyperinflated airways, as in emphysema.

Posterior percussion. Percuss across the top of each shoulder, then down toward the diaphragm at 2" (5-cm) intervals, comparing sounds on both sides as you proceed.

Lateral percussion. Ask the patient to raise his arms over his head. Percuss laterally at 2" (5-cm) intervals, comparing sounds on the right and left sides. Expect to hear resonance at these areas.

Diaphragmatic excursion. If you suspect a collapsed lung, measure the patient's diaphragmatic

excursion. Instruct the patient to take a deep breath and to hold it while you percuss downward, starting at the apex of the scapulae. Continue percussing downward until you hear dullness, indicating the lower border of the lung field. Mark this point. Ask him to exhale and hold his breath again as you percuss upward to the area of dullness. Mark this point, too. Repeat the procedure on the opposite side.

To calculate diaphragmatic excursion, measure the distance between the marks on each side. (Remember, the diaphragm's slightly higher on the right side.) Normal diaphragmatic excursion is about 2" to 2⅜" (5 to 6 cm) for a man; about 1⅛" to 2" (3 to 5 cm) for a woman. High resonance over the diaphragm may indicate pleural effusion or atelectasis.

PHYSICAL EXAMINATION CONTINUED

CHECKING FOR CARDIAC INVOLVEMENT

While monitoring your patient's vital signs, be prepared to run an EKG. The doctor may order this test to check for cardiac problems caused or exacerbated by the respiratory crisis. For example, if your patient has a preexisting dysrhythmia that increases his body's oxygen demand, an acute respiratory disorder could cause a *cardiac* crisis.

An EKG can also provide important clues about the respiratory disorder. For example, sinus tachycardia, a relatively minor dysrhythmia, may be the first sign of pulmonary embolism.

Cardiac conditions that may accompany a respiratory emergency include:

- supraventricular tachycardia
- atrial fibrillation
- ventricular irritability (possibly progressing to ventricular tachycardia).

The chart below shows which respiratory disorders may cause a specific dysrhythmia and describes each dysrhythmia's EKG features.

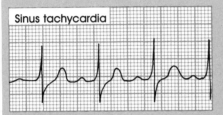

Sinus tachycardia

Respiratory cause
- Possibly the first sign of pulmonary embolism

EKG features and significance
- Rate is 100 to 160 beats/minute. (Tracing shows 130 beats/minute.)
- Impulse formation and conduction are normal.
- Prolonged sinus tachycardia may lead to ischemia and myocardial damage by raising oxygen requirements.

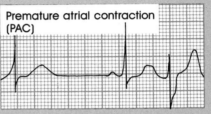

Premature atrial contraction (PAC)

Respiratory cause
- Acute respiratory failure or COPD

EKG features and significance
- Premature, occasionally abnormal P waves
- QRS complexes follow, except in very early or blocked PACs.
- P wave may be buried in the preceding T wave.
- Premature beat may be conducted aberrantly, as shown.

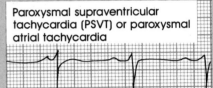

Paroxysmal supraventricular tachycardia (PSVT) or paroxysmal atrial tachycardia

Respiratory cause
- Hypoxia

EKG features and significance
- Heart rate > 140 beats/minute; rarely exceeds 250 beats/minute
- P waves are regular but aberrant; difficult to differentiate from preceding T wave.
- PSVT may cause palpitations, light-headedness, and exhaustion.

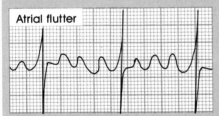

Atrial flutter

Respiratory cause
- Pulmonary embolism

EKG features and significance
- Ventricular rate (usually 60 to 100 beats/minute) depends on degree of AV block and is usually regular.
- Atrial rate is 250 to 400 beats/minute and usually regular.
- QRS complexes are uniform in shape; may be regular or irregular, depending on the degree of AV block.

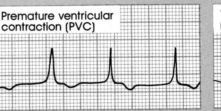

Premature ventricular contraction (PVC)

Respiratory cause
- Hypoxia, as in respiratory failure

EKG features and significance
- Focus can be unifocal (same appearance in every lead) or multifocal.
- Beat occurs prematurely, usually followed by a complete compensatory pause.
- QRS complex is wide (> 0.14 second) and distorted.
- Dysrhythmias can occur singly, in pairs, or in threes.

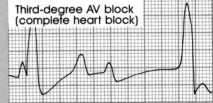

Third-degree AV block (complete heart block)

Respiratory cause
- Hypoxia

EKG features and significance
- Atrial impulses are blocked at AV node; atrial and ventricular impulses dissociated; no relationship between P waves and QRS complexes
- Atrial rate is regular; ventricular rate is slow and regular.
- Irregular PR interval.
- QRS interval may be normal or wide.

DIAGNOSTIC TESTS

DIAGNOSTIC TESTS: WHAT TO EXPECT

As you examine your patient in respiratory crisis, the doctor will order any or all of the following diagnostic tests.

Arterial blood gas (ABG) analysis. Expect the doctor to order ABG measurements immediately since this test requires only a blood specimen yet provides crucial diagnostic information. Although a specially trained nurse may perform the test, you'll be responsible for interpreting ABG measurements.

Pulmonary function tests. In most cases, you'll wait until the patient's airway is stable before calling a respiratory therapist to perform appropriate pulmonary function tests. However, you may need to measure the patient's vital capacity and tidal volume without waiting.

Thoracentesis. If the doctor suspects pleural effusion, he may order thoracentesis. (He may also perform this procedure to relieve increased lung pressure.)

Chest X-rays. If a portable X-ray machine's available, the doctor may order chest X-rays immediately. Assist the technician by positioning the patient.

To learn how to prepare for these and other diagnostic procedures, review the following pages.

ANALYZING pH BALANCE

If your patient's ABG measurements reveal acidosis or alkalosis, you can use his $PaCO_2$ and HCO_3^- values to determine whether the acid-base imbalance is caused by a respiratory or a metabolic problem. For example, if his pH level reveals acidosis, look for a $PaCO_2$ value greater than 45 mm Hg. Lung retention of CO_2 leads to respiratory acidosis—increased carbonic acid in the blood.

If his pH level shows alkalosis, look for a $PaCO_2$ value less than 35 mm Hg. Excessive expiration of CO_2 and water causes respiratory alkalosis—reduced carbonic acid in the blood.

Also, check to see if the lungs and kidneys—the principal acid-base regulators—have begun to compensate for the imbalance. Compensation may indicate a chronic disorder. For example, if the patient has respiratory acidosis, the kidneys gradually raise the blood's bicarbonate (base) level. In chronic metabolic acidosis, the lungs compensate by expiring more CO_2 and water, reducing the blood's carbonic acid level.

KEY TO A.B.G. ABBREVIATIONS

PaO
Partial pressure of oxygen in arterial blood.

PaCO
Partial pressure of carbon dioxide in arterial blood.

H₂CO
Carbonic acid (formed by carbon dioxide and water).

HCO ⁻
Bicarbonate (determined by a calculation involving pH and $PaCO_2$).

pH
Expression of hydrogen ion concentration.

SaO
Oxygen saturation (percentage of oxygen carried in hemoglobin).

REVIEWING A.B.G. ANALYSIS

The best diagnostic tool in a respiratory emergency, ABG analysis provides vital information about your patient's respiratory function within minutes. Based on blood specimens obtained from an arterial line or by percutaneous arterial puncture, this diagnostic test determines alveolar ventilation by measuring how much oxygen the lungs deliver to the blood (PaO_2) and how efficiently the lungs eliminate carbon dioxide ($PaCO_2$). It also measures blood pH, which may reveal acidosis or alkalosis. Comparing pH with $PaCO_2$, you can determine if your patient's acidosis or alkalosis stems from impaired gas exchange or a metabolic disorder.

While ABG analysis can distinguish a respiratory problem from a metabolic imbalance, it can't diagnose a specific pulmonary disease or differentiate a respiratory problem from a cardiac disorder. ABG analysis is most useful when correlated with measurements of ventilation and perfusion, cardiac output and tissue oxygenation, as well as findings from spirometry, chest X-ray, and other diagnostic tests.

Even though you probably won't have to obtain blood for an ABG test yourself, you'll probably have to interpret the results. Read on for guidelines on interpreting ABG measurements.

Note: If your patient's currently receiving medication, remember that certain drugs—for example, bicarbonates, hydrocortisones, chronically used laxatives, and thiazides—can increase his $PaCO_2$ level. Tetracycline, nitrofurazone (Furacin), methicillin sodium (Staphcillin), and acetazolamide (Diamox) can decrease his $PaCO_2$ level.

DIAGNOSTIC TESTS CONTINUED

INTERPRETING A.B.G. MEASUREMENTS

Do you know how to use an ABG analysis laboratory sheet to help you evaluate your patient's oxygenation, ventilation, and acid-base status? Use the chart below as a guide.

Oxygenation. PaO_2 and SaO_2 values reveal whether your patient's oxygen level is adequate. If he has mild hypoxemia, his PaO_2 level reveals the condition earlier than his SaO_2 value. In fact, PaO_2 can drop to as low as 50 mm Hg with no considerable change in SaO_2. However, SaO_2 will fall suddenly when PaO_2 drops below 50 mm Hg. *Note:* Abnormally low PaO_2 and SaO_2 values don't necessarily indicate hypoxemia. For example, an infant's PaO_2 is usually between 40 to 60 mm Hg; an elderly person's is usually below 80 mm Hg.

Ventilation. Does your patient have an abnormally high $PaCO_2$ value? Chances are he's hypo- ventilated and retained excessive CO_2 (hypercapnia). If his $PaCO_2$ value is abnormally low, he's hyperventilated and lost excessive CO_2 (hypocapnia).

Acid-base status. To find out if your patient's acidotic or alkalotic, see the information on page 35.

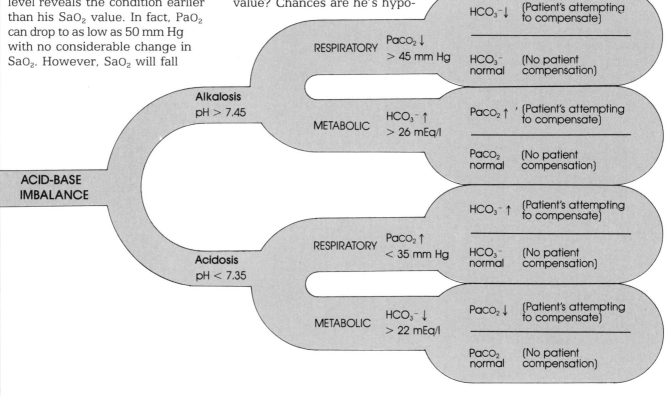

ACID-BASE IMBALANCE

Alkalosis
pH > 7.45

- RESPIRATORY $PaCO_2 \downarrow$ > 45 mm Hg
  - $HCO_3^- \downarrow$ (Patient's attempting to compensate)
  - HCO_3^- normal (No patient compensation)
- METABOLIC $HCO_3^- \uparrow$ > 26 mEq/l
  - $PaCO_2 \uparrow$ (Patient's attempting to compensate)
  - $PaCO_2$ normal (No patient compensation)

Acidosis
pH < 7.35

- RESPIRATORY $PaCO_2 \uparrow$ < 35 mm Hg
  - $HCO_3^- \uparrow$ (Patient's attempting to compensate)
  - HCO_3^- normal (No patient compensation)
- METABOLIC $HCO_3^- \downarrow$ > 22 mEq/l
  - $PaCO_2 \downarrow$ (Patient's attempting to compensate)
  - $PaCO_2$ normal (No patient compensation)

MEASURING A.B.G. VALUES: SOME NURSING CONSIDERATIONS

Is your patient scheduled for ABG testing? Keep these points in mind to help ensure valid test results and to reduce the risk of complications:
• Is your patient receiving oxygen? Check his chart to make sure he's been receiving the prescribed oxygen concentration for at least 15 minutes before obtaining a blood specimen. Document the liter flow on the laboratory slip.
• If the order specifies that he should be breathing room air, discontinue oxygen therapy 15 to 20 minutes before obtaining the specimen.
• The following factors can alter PaO_2 and $PaCO_2$ levels: exposing the specimen to air; failure to heparinize the syringe; and failure to send the specimen to the laboratory immediately.
• Is your patient receiving bicarbonates, ethacrynic acid, hydrocortisone, prednisone, or thiazides? These medications could increase his $PaCO_2$ level. Acetazolamide, methicillin, nitrofurantoin, and tetracycline may decrease his $PaCO_2$ level.
• After you've obtained the specimen, apply pressure to the puncture site and tape gauze over it. Monitor the patient's vital signs, and observe the site for bleeding, pain, swelling, discoloration, numbness, and tingling.

PULMONARY FUNCTION TESTS: EVALUATING VENTILATION

Pulmonary function tests evaluate respiratory function by measuring lung volume and capacity. Although some tests may not be performed during a crisis, they can be performed later to help identify the cause of the problem and to determine the degree of respiratory impairment. Pulmonary function tests can also help you monitor your patient's respiratory status and evaluate the effectiveness of his treatment.

Ventilatory function tests, one series of pulmonary function tests, measure the volume of air a patient inspires and expires during respiration, then estimate various lung capacities. These tests can also help distinguish between obstructive and restrictive ventilation defects.

Most pulmonary function tests use one of three techniques: diffusing spirometry, gas dilution and plethysmography, or diffusing capacity. (For all tests, you'll express the results as percentages, then compare them with predicted normal values based on the patient's age, height, and sex. Unless your patient has COPD, consider results abnormal if they're less than 80% of the predicted value.)

Spirometry. The most common pulmonary function study, spirometry is usually the first test performed. During a complete spirometry test, which is usually done in a pulmonary function laboratory, the patient breathes through a mouthpiece attached to a machine (spirometer) that measures and records seven pulmonary function indices: tidal volume, expiratory reserve volume, vital capacity, inspiratory capacity, forced vital capacity (FVC), forced expiratory volume (FEV), and maximal voluntary ventilation. These measurements can be used to calculate other pulmonary function measurements, such as functional residual capacity, total lung capacity, and maximal midexpiratory flow.

Using FVC and FEV, you may be able to distinguish between restrictive and obstructive lung disorders. For instance, while decreased FVC and FEV may

---

Some sedatives and narcotic analgesics can interfere with pulmonary function tests. Check with the doctor.

---

both indicate a restrictive disorder, FEV is reduced less than FVC in a restrictive disease. (This disease type doesn't change airway resistance.)

Depending on the situation, you may have instruments at hand that enable you or a respiratory therapist to perform an abbreviated spirometry test immediately. With a bedside spirometer, you can measure your patient's FVC and FEV; using a peak flowmeter, you can measure how fast air flows in and out of his lungs during respiration.

Gas dilution and plethysmography. During a gas dilution test, the patient breathes a measured amount of relatively insoluble gas, such as helium, that's mixed with oxygen in a closed system. The gas dilution in the breathing mixture is then analyzed. Gas dilution permits a more precise calculation of pulmonary functions, such as residual volume, total lung capacity, and functional residual capacity. Because it differentiates restrictive from obstructive disease more reliably than spirometry, the gas dilution test can be used to confirm spirometry findings.

But if the diagnosis requires more precise information, the doctor may order plethysmography. For this test, the patient's sealed in an airtight glass container while a machine measures and records gas volumes, airway resistance, and alveolar pressure.

Diffusing capacity. If other pulmonary function tests or ABG measurements reveal abnormal ventilation, evaluating the patient's diffusing capacity for carbon monoxide will help determine whether the disorder has impaired gas exchange across the respiratory membrane. This easily performed test identifies and evaluates diffusion defects by measuring the rate at which a highly soluble gas, such as carbon monoxide, passes through the respiratory membrane.

The patient first exhales, then deeply inhales a measured concentration of carbon monoxide. After holding his breath for about 10 seconds to allow the gas to diffuse, he exhales into a rubber bag. Gas transfer is determined by comparing the inhaled and exhaled gas concentrations.

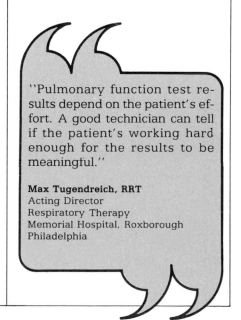

"Pulmonary function test results depend on the patient's effort. A good technician can tell if the patient's working hard enough for the results to be meaningful."

Max Tugendreich, RRT
Acting Director
Respiratory Therapy
Memorial Hospital, Roxborough
Philadelphia

DIAGNOSTIC TESTS CONTINUED

INTERPRETING PULMONARY FUNCTION TESTS

PULMONARY FUNCTION MEASUREMENT	CALCULATION METHOD	IMPLICATIONS
Tidal volume (V_T)—average amount of air inhaled or exhaled during normal breathing	Determine the spirographic measurement for 10 breaths, then divide by 10.	Decreased V_T may indicate restrictive disease and requires further testing.
Minute volume—total amount of air breathed per minute	Multiply V_T by the respiratory rate.	Normal minute volume can occur in emphysema; decreased minute volume may indicate other diseases.
Inspiratory capacity (IC)—amount of air that can be inhaled after normal expiration	Direct spirographic measurement; or add inspiratory reserve volume (IRV) and V_T.	Decreased IC indicates restrictive disease.
Inspiratory reserve volume (IRV)—amount of air inspired beyond normal inspiration	Subtract V_T from IC.	Abnormal IRV alone doesn't indicate respiratory dysfunction; IRV decreases during normal exercise.
Expiratory reserve volume (ERV)—amount of air that can be exhaled after normal expiration	Direct spirographic measurement.	ERV varies, even in healthy persons.
Residual volume (RV)—amount of air remaining in the lungs after forced expiration	Subtract ERV from functional residual capacity (FRC).	RV greater than 35% of total lung capacity (TLC) after maximal expiratory effort may indicate obstructive disease.
Vital capacity (VC)—total volume of air that can be exhaled after maximum inspiration	Direct spirographic measurement; or add V_T, IRV, and ERV.	Normal or increased VC with decreased flow rates may indicate reduction in functional pulmonary tissue. Decreased VC with normal or increased flow rates may indicate decreased respiratory effort.
Functional residual capacity (FRC)—amount of air remaining in the lungs after normal expiration	Helium dilution technique measurement; or add ERV and RV.	Increased FRC indicates overdistention of lungs, which may result from obstructive pulmonary disease. Decreased FRC indicates restrictive lung disease.
Total lung capacity (TLC)—total volume of the lungs when maximally inflated	Add V_T, IRV, ERV, and RV; or FRC and IC; or VC and RV.	Low TLC indicates restrictive lung disease; high TLC indicates overdistended lungs associated with obstructive disease.
Forced vital capacity (FVC)—measurement of the amount of air quickly and forcefully exhaled after maximum inspiration	Direct spirographic measurement at 1-, 2-, and 3-second intervals.	Decreased FVC indicates flow resistance in the respiratory system from an obstructive disease.
Forced expiratory volume (FEV)—volume of air expired in 1st, 2nd, or 3rd second of FVC maneuver	Direct spirographic measurement; expressed as percentage of FVC.	Decreased FEV_1 and increased FEV_2 and FEV_3 may indicate obstructive disease; decreased or normal FEV_1 may indicate restrictive disease.

REVIEWING THORACENTESIS

If you find signs of pleural effusion, pneumothorax, or hemothorax during palpation and percussion, the doctor may perform thoracentesis to diagnose and treat the patient.

Normally, the pleural space contains less than 20 ml of serous fluid. If pleural fluid forms abnormally or isn't properly absorbed, it accumulates in the pleural space, causing pleural effusion.

Thoracentesis, a fluid-draining procedure, relieves pulmonary compression and its resulting respiratory distress. To diagnose the cause of the effusion, the doctor analyzes the fluid for color, consistency, glucose and protein content, cellular composition, and presence of the enzymes lactic dehydrogenase and amylase. For example, blood-tinged fluid indicates hemothorax; milky fluid indicates traumatic rupture of the thoracic duct. Low-protein fluid—fluid leaked from normal vessels—is classified as transudate fluid. It usually indicates cirrhosis or congestive heart failure.

Protein-rich fluid—leaked from highly permeable blood vessels—is referred to as exudate fluid. This type of fluid is found in infectious disease, asbestosis, pulmonary infarction, or lymphatic drainage disorders.

Read on for instructions on how to assist the doctor before and after thoracentesis.

Preparing the patient. Before thoracentesis, explain the procedure to the patient. Warn him that he may experience a stinging sensation when the doctor injects the anesthetic and that he'll feel pressure as the doctor withdraws the pleural fluid.

Record his vital signs, then place him in one of the following three positions:
• seated on the edge of the bed, with his feet resting on a stool or chair and his arms on an overbed table
• seated in bed with his head and arms resting on several pillows stacked on an overbed table
• lying on his unaffected side, with the arm on the affected side elevated above his head.
These positions widen the intercostal spaces and permit easy access to the pleural cavity.

Advise the patient not to cough, breathe deeply, or move suddenly during the test, to avoid the risk of internal damage.

Post-test care. Record the patient's vital signs. Then reposition him comfortably on the affected side (or as ordered by the doctor). Tell him to remain in this position for at least 1 hour, to seal the puncture site.

Watch him closely for signs and symptoms of the following complications:
• Pneumothorax. Check for apprehension, cyanosis, or sudden breathlessness.
• Tension pneumothorax. Monitor him for chest pain, tachycardia, or absent or diminished breath sounds on the affected side.
• Fluid reaccumulation. Check for increasing and persistent cough or respiratory distress.
• Mediastinal shift. Check for labored breathing, cardiac distress, or pulmonary edema (pink frothy sputum, paradoxical pulse).

Documentation. On the patient's chart, document the color and amount of pleural fluid obtained, and indicate which studies the doctor ordered. Also note how well the patient tolerated the procedure.

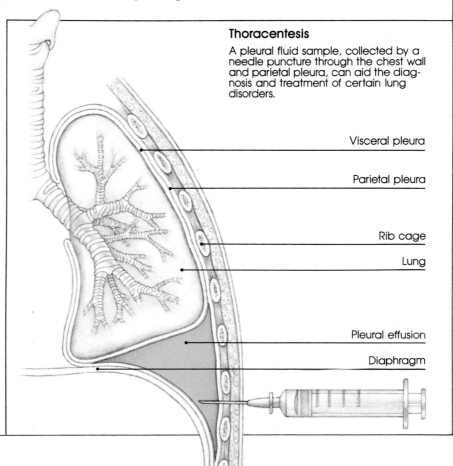

Thoracentesis

A pleural fluid sample, collected by a needle puncture through the chest wall and parietal pleura, can aid the diagnosis and treatment of certain lung disorders.

Visceral pleura

Parietal pleura

Rib cage

Lung

Pleural effusion

Diaphragm

DIAGNOSTIC TESTS CONTINUED

SIGNIFICANCE OF PLEURAL FLUID ANALYSIS

GRAM STAIN CULTURE AND SENSITIVITY

Interpretation
A positive result may indicate early stages of bacterial infection. In later stages of infection, fluid may appear grossly purulent with a positive Gram stain, yet cultures may be negative from antibiotic therapy.

ACID-FAST STAIN AND CULTURE

Interpretation
A positive result may indicate tuberculosis.

RED BLOOD CELL COUNT

Interpretation
A count of about 10,000/mm³ in a pink or light-red specimen may indicate tissue damage. A count above 100,000/mm³ in a grossly bloody specimen may suggest pulmonary infarction or closed chest trauma. If a hemothorax is present, pleural fluid hematocrit will resemble that of capillary blood.

LEUKOCYTE COUNT

Interpretation
A count above 1,000/mm³ or over 50% neutrophils may indicate septic or nonseptic inflammation.

BLOOD CLOTS

Interpretation
May indicate neoplasm, tuberculosis, or infection.

SPECIFIC GRAVITY

Interpretation
A measurement exceeding 1.016 may indicate neoplasm, tuberculosis, or infection; a measurement less than 1.104 may indicate congestive heart failure.

TOTAL PROTEIN

Interpretation
A level below 3 g/dl may indicate a transudative disorder.
A level above 3 g/dl may suggest infection.

LACTIC DEHYDROGENASE

Interpretation
Levels rise in exudative disorders; levels decrease in transudative disorders.

GLUCOSE

Interpretation
A level lower than the serum glucose level may suggest bacterial infection or nonseptic inflammation.

SEDIMENT

Interpretation
May represent cellular debris or cholesterol crystals.

CHEST X-RAYS AND OTHER RADIOLOGIC TESTS

During any respiratory emergency, the doctor will order chest X-rays. Almost as routine as ABG measurements, chest X-rays can:
• detect and evaluate lung disorders, such as pneumonia, atelectasis, pneumothorax, pulmonary blebs, and tumors
• determine the size and location of a lesion
• indicate the correct placement of an endotracheal tube
• distinguish pulmonary edema from lung inflammation and infection. (However, this requires a special procedure—the gravitational shift test—that uses gravity and serial X-rays.)

When are chest X-rays unreliable? They may appear normal in patients with bronchial asthma, chronic bronchitis, and early or intermediate stages of emphysema. Chest X-rays may also be normal in respiratory insufficiency stemming from any of the following disorders:
• extrapulmonary abnormality, such as brain and spinal cord damage (unless pulmonary infection is present)
• neuromuscular disorder (for example, poliomyelitis or myasthenia gravis)
• respiratory depression caused by a sedative overdose.

In such cases, accurate diagnosis may require additional radiologic tests. Read the chart on the following page to learn more about these tests.

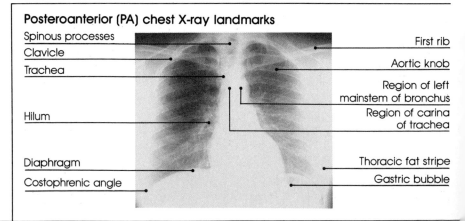

Posteroanterior (PA) chest X-ray landmarks

Spinous processes
Clavicle
Trachea
Hilum
Diaphragm
Costophrenic angle

First rib
Aortic knob
Region of left mainstem of bronchus
Region of carina of trachea
Thoracic fat stripe
Gastric bubble

RECOGNIZING ABNORMAL X-RAY FINDINGS

NORMAL ANATOMIC LOCATION AND APPEARANCE	ABNORMALITY	POSSIBLE RESPIRATORY IMPLICATIONS
Trachea Visible midline in the anterior mediastinal cavity; translucent; tubelike	• Deviation from midline	• Tension pneumothorax, atelectasis, pleural effusion
Heart Visible in the left anterior mediastinal cavity; solid appearance from blood contents; edges may be clear in contrast to the surrounding air density of the lung	• Shift • Hypertrophy of right heart • Cardiac borders obscured by stringy densities ("shaggy heart")	• Atelectasis • Cor pulmonale • Cystic fibrosis
Mediastinum (mediastinal shadow) Visible as a space between the lungs; shadowy appearance that widens at the hilum	• Deviation to the nondiseased side; deviation toward the diseased side by traction • Gross widening	• Pleural effusion of tumor, fibrosis, or collapsed lung • Neoplasms of bronchi or lungs; mediastinitis; cor pulmonale
Ribs Visible as thoracic cavity encasement	• Break or misalignment • Widening of intercostal spaces	• Fractured sternum or ribs • Emphysema
Clavicles Visible in upper thorax; intact and equidistant in properly centered X-ray films	• Break or misalignment	• Fractures
Hila (lung roots) Visible where bronchi join the lungs; appear as small, white, bilateral densities	• Shift to one side • Accentuated shadows	• Atelectasis • Emphysema, pulmonary abscess
Mainstem bronchus Visible to about 1" (2.5 cm) from hila; translucent; tubelike	• Spherical or oval density	• Bronchogenic cyst
Bronchi Usually not visible	• Visible	• Bronchial pneumonia
Lung fields Usually not visible throughout, except for fine white areas from the hilum	• Visible • Irregular, patchy densities	• Atelectasis • Resolving pneumonia, silicosis, fibrosis
Hemidiaphragm Rounded, visible; right side ⅜" to ¾" (1 to 2 cm) higher than left	• Elevation of diaphragm • Flattening of diaphragm • Unilateral elevation of either side	• Pneumonia, pleurisy, acute bronchitis, atelectasis • Asthma, emphysema • Pneumothorax or pulmonary infection

DIAGNOSTIC TESTS CONTINUED

OTHER DIAGNOSTIC TESTS: RADIOLOGIC PROCEDURES

NONINVASIVE TESTS

Radiologic test	Description	Diagnostic purpose
Fluoroscopy	An image intensifier passes a stream of X-rays through the patient, projecting a continuous image of thoracic structures to a fluorescent screen.	• Detects bronchiolar obstruction and pulmonary disease by measuring lung expansion and contraction during quiet breathing, deep breathing, and coughing; and by showing diaphragmatic movement • Defines location and movement of mediastinal lesions during breathing and swallowing more precisely than do X-rays
Ultrasonography (A-mode presentation)	A transducer beams sound waves cross-sectionally through the body, converting reflected sound to electrical impulses and producing a thoracic image on an oscilloscope.	• Detects pleural effusion and defines the effusion's boundaries when chest X-ray and thoracentesis fail • Determines whether mediastinal and near-chest-wall lesions are fluid or solid

INVASIVE TESTS

Radiologic test	Description	Diagnostic purpose
Pulmonary angiography	Radiopaque iodine contrast medium, inserted into the pulmonary artery or one of its branches, produces an X-ray showing pulmonary circulation.	• Detects and conclusively confirms pulmonary embolism • Identifies lung tissue changes, such as tumors and blebs • Identifies defects in pulmonary vascular perfusion, such as aneurysms, vessel displacement, and diminished blood flow • Measures pressure at various sites during catheter insertion
Ventilation scanning	A nuclear scan, performed after the patient inhales air mixed with radioactive gas, delineates lung areas ventilated during respiration. Gas distribution is recorded during three phases: inspiration, maximum concentration, and expiration.	• Helps diagnose pulmonary embolism • Evaluates regional respiratory function; locates regional hypoventilation, usually caused by chronic obstructive pulmonary disease or excessive smoking
Lung perfusion scan (called lung scintigraphy when used with ventilation scan)	Inhaled or I.V.-injected radiopaque contrast medium produces a visual image of pulmonary blood flow.	• Identifies pulmonary vascular obstructions, such as pulmonary embolism • When results are compared with ventilation findings, shows ventilation-perfusion patterns

VENTILATION PROBLEMS

ACUTE RESPIRATORY FAILURE

AIRWAY OBSTRUCTION

ARTIFICIAL AIRWAYS

SPECIAL PROBLEMS

C.O.P.D. BASICS

C.O.P.D. ASSESSMENT

C.O.P.D. MANAGEMENT

RESTRICTIVE
LUNG DISEASE

PLEURAL EFFUSION

ATELECTASIS

PNEUMONIA

RELATED CRISES

ACUTE RESPIRATORY FAILURE

A.R.F.: CRISIS WITH MANY CAUSES

Doris Mulligan, a 32-year-old realtor, is recovering from severe head injuries she suffered in a car accident. As you monitor her condition for complications, watch for signs of acute respiratory failure (ARF)—even though her lungs are uninjured.

To understand why, consider this working definition of ARF: insufficient blood oxygenation and/or CO_2 removal, regardless of the cause. An emergency that can develop rapidly or over several days, ARF can succeed various conditions—with or without underlying lung disease.

Although in some patients ARF complicates chronic bronchitis, asthma, or emphysema, it can also strike when lung tissue is essentially healthy; for example, as a complication of myocardial infarction, congestive heart failure, pulmonary embolism, or any injury or condition that impairs ventilation. And, because head injuries may impair the brain's respiratory control center, a patient like Ms. Mulligan is at risk, too.

Pathophysiology. Four abnormal mechanisms—alveolar hypoventilation, intrapulmonary shunting, ventilation/perfusion mismatch, and impaired diffusion across the respiratory membrane—can impair gas exchange in ARF. Two or more of these mechanisms may operate simultaneously.

Regardless of the underlying mechanism, impaired gas exchange ultimately affects the entire body. Along with the respiratory system, the brain, kidneys, heart, and blood vessels undergo compensatory changes. Without medical intervention, however, adequate oxygenation can't be restored.

Common denominators. What do all ARF victims have in common? Hypoxia and/or hypercapnia, the twin hallmarks of ARF. As a rule, arterial blood gas (ABG) values provide the key. For most patients, an arterial oxygen (PaO_2) level below 50 mm Hg or an arterial carbon dioxide ($PaCO_2$) level above 50 mm Hg indicates ARF.

Like most rules, however, this one has exceptions. It doesn't apply to patients with chronic obstructive pulmonary disease (COPD), because they have chronically low PaO_2 values and high $PaCO_2$ values. For them, any sudden or extreme shift in baseline values suggests ARF.

ARF types. Although various problems can contribute to ARF, we can classify the condition into two general categories: those caused primarily by *ventilation impairment* and those caused by *oxygenation disorders*. In ventilation impairment, oxygen can't reach the alveoli because of a transport problem; for example, an upper airway obstruction. In an oxygenation disorder, oxygen reaches the alveoli but isn't absorbed or utilized properly. For examples of each ARF type, see the box below.

In the remainder of this section, we'll discuss the three kinds of ventilation impairment: upper airway obstruction, COPD, and restrictive lung disease. Then, in Section 4, we'll examine oxygenation disorders.

You'll note that we've devoted Section 5 to trauma-related ARF. Although chest trauma can induce either type of respiratory failure, this emergency requires specialized intervention, which we'll consider separately.

CLASSIFYING A.R.F.

Although ARF isn't itself a disease, it's a potential end result of many disease conditions—several of which may occur simultaneously. Conditions impairing ventilation initially produce hypercapnia; those impairing oxygenation produce hypoxia. Read what follows for some common examples.

IMPAIRED VENTILATION

• Anaphylaxis
• Asthma
• Atelectasis
• Bronchitis
• Drug overdose (for example, of barbiturates or sedatives)
• Emphysema
• Fractures (especially of the ribs)
• Guillain-Barré syndrome
• Myasthenia gravis
• Pleural effusion
• Pneumonia
• Pneumothorax
• Thoracic surgery or trauma
• Upper airway obstruction (for example, by the tongue or a foreign body)

IMPAIRED OXYGENATION

• Adult respiratory distress syndrome (ARDS)
• Aspiration of acids or bile
• Lung tumors
• Near drowning
• Pulmonary emboli
• Pulmonary edema
• Toxic chemical inhalation

YOUR PATIENT'S RESPONSE

Although ABG values are the most reliable diagnostic indicators of ARF, don't underestimate the value of your assessment skills for spotting a developing problem. The hypoxia and hypercapnia characteristic of ARF stimulate strong responses by the respiratory, cardiovascular, and central nervous systems. Here's how each system's affected—and what you should watch for.

Respiratory response. When the body senses hypoxia or hypercapnia (or both), the brain's respiratory center responds by first increasing respiratory depth (tidal volume); then, respiratory rate. As a result, your patient hyperventilates. This and any other sign of labored breathing—flared nostrils, pursed-lip exhalation, and use of accessory breathing muscles—portend ARF. As respiratory failure worsens, you'll probably see intercostal, supraclavicular, and suprasternal retractions, too.

Cardiovascular response. As a rule, the sympathetic nervous system responds to an emergency such as hypoxia by increasing the heart rate and constricting blood vessels. Besides helping to raise blood pressure and cardiac output, vasoconstriction makes your patient's skin cool, pale, and clammy.

But high $PaCO_2$ can have an opposite effect on smooth muscle vessels, causing peripheral vasodilation. Instead of appearing cool and clammy, your patient's skin may feel warm and flushed. If this opposing effect outweighs normal sympathetic vasoconstriction, blood pressure may drop—possibly leading to shock.

Because cardiovascular symptoms are variable, your best indicator is any significant *change* in vital signs.

Central nervous system response. Even a slight disruption in oxygen supply and carbon dioxide removal affects brain function—and, in turn, your patient's behavior. Brain hypoxia and rising $PaCO_2$ levels can cause restlessness or lethargy, irritability, anxiety, depression, and confusion.

Don't depend on cyanosis to warn you of hypoxia. By the time it's apparent, your patient may be in crisis.

The patient may also develop a headache, as cerebral vessels dilate in an effort to increase the brain's blood supply. In addition, high $PaCO_2$ levels may cause his muscles to twitch and his arms and legs to tingle. If $PaCO_2$ levels continue to rise, he may develop convulsions and become comatose.

From failure to arrest. If ARF progresses to respiratory arrest, every moment counts; without adequate ventilation, the body depletes arterial oxygen in seconds. After only 6 minutes without oxygen, the brain suffers irreversible damage.

When respiratory arrest precedes cardiac arrest, the patient's heart may beat for several more minutes. His chest may continue to move slightly, although ventilation is negligible. His level of consciousness diminishes greatly, although he may respond purposelessly to stimulation. His pale or cyanotic skin reflects systemic hypoxia.

If the patient's in total respiratory arrest, he completely loses consciousness, and chest or abdominal movement ceases. You won't be able to detect airflow or expiratory sounds from his upper airway.

In such a case, immediately begin cardiopulmonary resuscitation, following accepted procedures. Read the following pages for details on how to proceed if an upper airway obstruction causes respiratory arrest.

Assessment findings in ARF

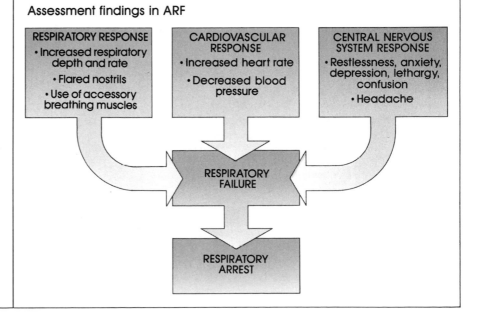

RESPIRATORY RESPONSE	CARDIOVASCULAR RESPONSE	CENTRAL NERVOUS SYSTEM RESPONSE
• Increased respiratory depth and rate • Flared nostrils • Use of accessory breathing muscles	• Increased heart rate • Decreased blood pressure	• Restlessness, anxiety, depression, lethargy, confusion • Headache

RESPIRATORY FAILURE

RESPIRATORY ARREST

AIRWAY OBSTRUCTION

AIRWAY OBSTRUCTION: ACT FAST

Few sights are more frightening than a patient clutching his throat, unable to speak. These classic signs of upper airway obstruction signal the need for immediate intervention. Without ventilation, his body uses up its arterial oxygen supply within a few seconds. Irreversible brain damage follows within 6 minutes.

Causes and intervention. A variety of problems can cause upper airway obstruction, including:
• aspiration of a foreign object, blood, mucus, or vomitus
• tongue relaxation over the hypopharynx
• edema of the larynx or vocal cords from anaphylaxis, neck trauma, or acute epiglottitis.

Regardless of the cause, you'll respond to this respiratory emergency by attempting to clear the airway and restore breathing. (Beginning on this page, we provide guidelines.) If you're unsuccessful, prepare to assist with endotracheal intubation, cricothyrotomy, or tracheotomy.

Headed for trouble. The signs of complete airway obstruction are unmistakable. But signs and symptoms of partial or impending airway obstruction are distinctive, too. Watch for these warning signs: stridor on inspiration; exaggerated chest movements; muffled voice sounds; ashen, pallid, or cyanotic skin color; nostril flaring; tachycardia; restlessness, agitation, and anxiety.

Caution: Breathing difficulties and respiratory arrest can result from problems other than airway obstruction; for example, respiratory paralysis from a central nervous system disorder or overoxygenation. Provide respiratory support and take other action appropriate to the underlying cause.

CLEARING A CONSCIOUS PATIENT'S AIRWAY

Your patient, who's clutching her throat and has her mouth open, is exhibiting the universal sign of airway obstruction.

Immediately ask her if she can speak. If she answers—or if she coughs and chokes—her airway's partially open. Stand by and provide reassurance, but don't interfere. She may be able to clear her airway by herself.

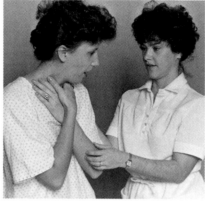

If she can't speak—or if you note extreme breathing difficulty, stridor, weak or ineffective cough, or cyanosis—intervene immediately. Stand behind her and support her with one arm. If possible, position her head below her shoulders to take advantage of gravitational force. Then cup your hand and deliver four sharp blows over her spine between the scapulae.

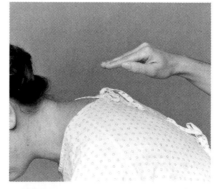

If these measures aren't effective, perform abdominal thrusts. Standing behind the patient, wrap both arms around her waist. Place your fist in the center of her abdomen, midway between the umbilicus and the xiphoid process. Rest the thumb side of your fist against her epigastrium. Then, grasp your fist with your other hand. Using a quick motion, thrust your fists inward and upward four times.

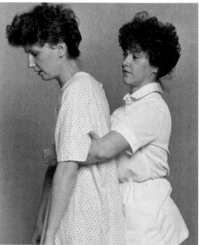

Alternate back blows with abdominal thrusts until you clear the airway or the patient loses consciousness. *Note:* Don't continue to give abdominal thrusts if a previous thrust has cleared the airway.

If the patient loses consciousness, ease him to the floor and call for help. In the following photostory, we demonstrate how to clear an unconscious patient's airway.

WHEN YOUR PATIENT'S UNCONSCIOUS

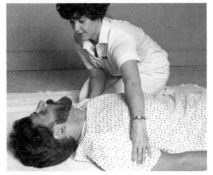

1 You discover a patient who's collapsed unconscious beside his bed. Your first step is to try rousing him.

To do this, and still protect yourself from injury, firmly grasp his upper arms, as the nurse is doing here. This limits his range of motion if his arms begin to flail. Then shake him and call his name.
Caution: Don't shake him vigorously if you suspect spinal damage or any other serious injury.

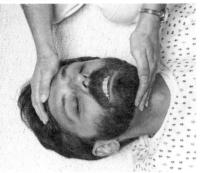

2 No response? Call for help, and position the patient flat on his back. Open his airway with the *head-tilt/chin-lift method.* Place your hand that's closest to the patient's head on his forehead, and tilt his head slightly back. Place the fingertips of your other hand under his lower jaw, on the bony part near his chin. Gently lift up his chin, taking care not to close his mouth. *Note:* If you suspect a neck injury, don't tilt his neck (see photo 12 for guidelines).

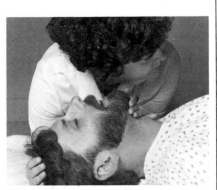

3 Now check for restored breathing. Position your ear slightly above his mouth and nose. Listen for breath sounds, feel for air movement against your cheek, and watch his chest and abdomen for movement.

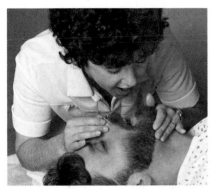

4 Attempt to ventilate, as the nurse is doing here. If this isn't successful, reposition the patient's airway and try to ventilate again. If your second attempt doesn't succeed, assume his airway is blocked.

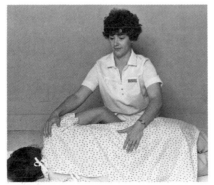

5 Logroll the patient toward you, and brace your thigh against his chest.

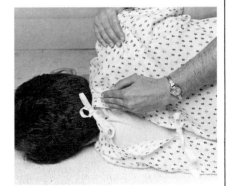

6 With a cupped hand, deliver four sharp back blows between his scapulae.

CONTINUED ON PAGE 48

ARTIFICIAL AIRWAYS CONTINUED

WHEN YOUR PATIENT'S UNCONSCIOUS CONTINUED

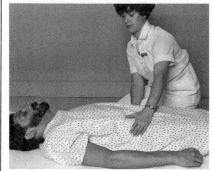

7 Now, roll the patient onto his back. Depending on your size and the size of the patient, either kneel astride his hips or at his side.

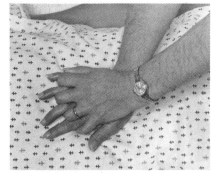

8 Lace your fingers together, and place the heel of your bottom hand over the epigastrium (above the umbilicus but below the xiphoid process). With four quick thrusts, press the heel of your bottom hand inward and upward (toward the patient's head).

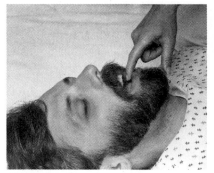

9 Open his mouth by pulling down his lower lip, and look for an obstructing object or substance.

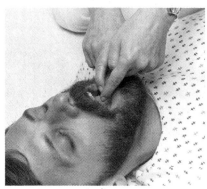

10 If the obstruction's visible, attempt to remove it using the finger-sweep method. Then reposition his head and attempt to ventilate him. Continue to deliver back blows, abdominal thrusts, and rescue breaths until breathing's restored or a tracheotomy becomes necessary.

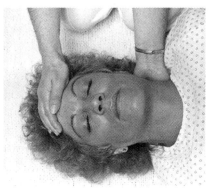

11 As an alternative, you can use the *head-tilt/neck-lift* method. Place one hand on the patient's forehead and the other under her neck, close to the back of her head. Gently press back on her forehead while lifting and supporting her neck.

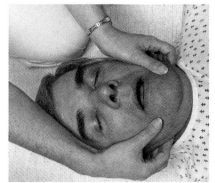

12 If you suspect the patient has a spinal injury, use the *jaw-thrust* method. Kneel at his head, facing his feet. Place your thumbs on his jaw near the corners of his mouth, pointing your thumbs toward his feet. Then, position the tips of your index fingers at the angles of his jaw. As the nurse is demonstrating in this photo, push your thumbs down while you lift upward with the tips of your index fingers.

PERFORMING CHEST THRUSTS

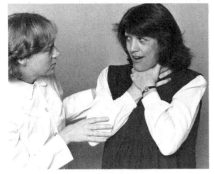

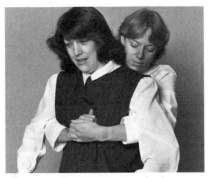

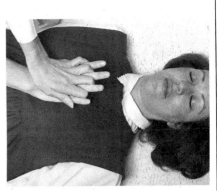

1 If your patient's pregnant, abdominal thrusts are contra-indicated. And if she's obese, abdominal thrusts may not clear an airway obstruction. For such patients (and for children), use chest thrusts instead.

2 If your patient's conscious and upright, stand behind her and wrap your arms around her, directly under her armpits. Make a fist, placing your thumb over the third phlange of your index finger. Align your thumb with the patient's sternum, then grab your fist with the opposite hand. Next, press against the sternum forcefully with four quick thrusts.

3 If your patient's unconscious and supine, position yourself at her side as you would to deliver chest compressions. (Or, if you can comfortably do so, kneel astride her hips.) Position your hands as you would to give chest compressions, on the lower portion of her sternum. (But take care to avoid her xiphoid process.) Thrust inward and upward (toward her head) four times.

HOW TO USE A HAND-HELD RESUSCITATOR

In a hospital, you won't have to ventilate a patient with mouth-to-mouth ventilation for long. Instead, you'll continue life-saving measures as necessary with a hand-held resuscitator, such as an Ambu bag. But using it properly requires some guidelines. To ensure effective ventilation:

Make sure you have enough room to work. Remove the bed's headboard if possible, and move the bed away from the wall. Position yourself behind the patient's head.

First, attach the mask to the bag. Then hyperextend the patient's neck and place the mask over his face. Position the mask so the apex of the triangle is over the bridge of the nose and the base is between the lower lip and chin. (See photo at right.)

Hold the mask in place with

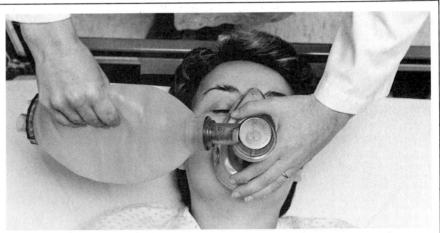

your nondominant hand to create a tight seal. Exert firm pressure to maintain neck hyperextension and to hold the mask in place. Use your other hand to squeeze the bag and to operate suction equipment, if necessary, between breaths. Squeeze the bag approximately once every 5 seconds for an adult (once every 3 seconds for an infant).

Watch for the patient's chest to rise and fall and for the bag to deflate completely with each squeeze. Don't worry if air's escaping around the mask as long as you see these two signs that you're providing adequate ventilation.

Note: Attach an oxygen line to the resuscitator as necessary.

ARTIFICIAL AIRWAYS

COMPARING ARTIFICIAL AIRWAYS

When a patient's threatened by an upper airway obstruction, inserting an artificial airway may be one of your first priorities. But choosing an *appropriate* airway depends on several factors, including the patient's condition. This chart details the points to consider before taking action.

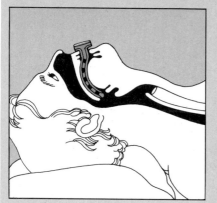

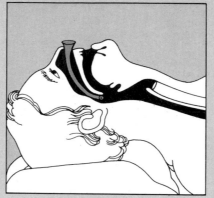

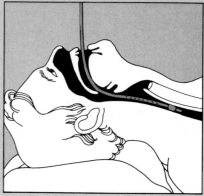

OROPHARYNGEAL

Indications
• Airway obstruction, when nasopharyngeal airway is contraindicated because of nasal obstruction or predisposition to epistaxis
• Short-term intubation

Contraindications
• Trauma to lower face
• Oral surgery

Advantages
• Easily inserted
• Holds tongue away from pharynx

Disadvantages
• Dislodges easily
• May stimulate gag reflex
• May cause obstruction if airway size is incorrect
• Poorly tolerated by most conscious patients

NASOPHARYNGEAL

Indications
• Airway obstruction, when oropharyngeal airway is contraindicated because of trauma to lower face or oral surgery
• Surgery, to maintain patent airway until patient recovers from anesthesia

Contraindications
• Nasal obstruction
• Predisposition to epistaxis

Advantages
• Easily inserted
• Tolerated better than oropharyngeal airway by conscious patients
• Allows for suctioning without displacing the patient's nasal turbinates

Disadvantages
• May cause severe epistaxis if inserted too forcefully
• May kink and clog, obstructing airway
• May cause pressure necrosis of nasal mucosa
• May cause air passage obstruction, if artificial airway is too large

ORAL ESOPHAGEAL

Indication
• Airway obstruction, when all other efforts to maintain an open airway have failed (used primarily in emergency departments or by trained paramedics)

Contraindications
• Trauma to lower face
• Oral surgery

Advantages
• Quickly and easily inserted
• Prevents aspiration of stomach contents while tube is in place

Disadvantages
• May cause pharyngeal trauma during insertion
• May be accidentally inserted into trachea
• May cause gastric distension and may impair ventilation if cuff is improperly inflated

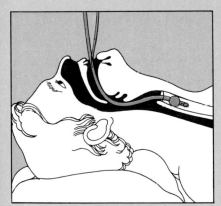 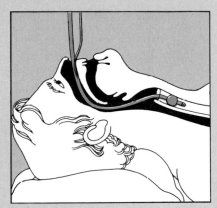 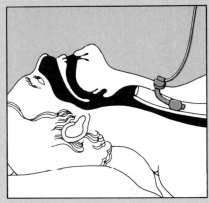

ORAL ENDOTRACHEAL

Indications
• Cardiopulmonary resuscitation or other airway obstruction, when all other efforts to maintain an open airway have failed and when patient has nasal obstruction or predisposition to epistaxis
• Mechanical ventilation, when patient has nasal obstruction or predisposition to epistaxis
• Short-term intubation

Contraindications
• Trauma to lower face
• Oral surgery
• Long-term intubation

Advantages
• Quickly and easily inserted
• Causes less intubation trauma than nasal endotracheal airway or trach tube
• Prevents aspiration of stomach contents, if cuff is inflated

Disadvantages
• May damage teeth or lacerate lips, mouth, pharyngeal mucosa, or larynx during insertion
• Activates gag reflex in conscious patients
• Kinks and clogs easily
• May be bitten or chewed
• May cause pressure necrosis, middle-ear infection, laryngeal edema, or tracheal damage

NASAL ENDOTRACHEAL

Indications
• Airway obstruction, when all other efforts to maintain an open airway have failed and when patient has facial trauma
• Mechanical ventilation
• Long-term intubation

Contraindications
• Nasal obstruction
• Fractured nose
• Sinusitis
• Predisposition to epistaxis

Advantages
• More comfortable than oral endotracheal tube
• Permits good oral hygiene
• Can't be bitten or chewed
• Provides a channel for suctioning
• May be adapted easily if patient requires continuous ventilation
• Can be anchored in place easily
• Prevents aspiration of stomach contents, if cuff is inflated

Disadvantages
• May lacerate pharyngeal mucosa or layrnx during insertion
• Kinks and clogs easily
• Increases airway resistance because of small lumen size needed to fit nasal passages
• May cause pressure necrosis, middle-ear infection, laryngeal edema, or tracheal damage

TRACHEOSTOMY

Indications
• Complete upper airway obstruction, when endotracheal intubation is impossible
• Long-term intubation

Contraindications
• Whenever patient's highly susceptible to infection; for example, when he's receiving an immunosuppressant drug
• Short-term intubation

Advantages
• Suctioned more easily than endotracheal tube
• Reduces dead air space in respiratory tract
• Causes less trauma to airways
• Permits patient to swallow and eat more easily
• More comfortable than other tubes
• Prevents aspiration of stomach contents, if cuff is inflated

Disadvantages
• Requires surgery to insert
• May cause laceration or pressure necrosis of trachea
• May cause tracheoesophageal fistula
• Increases risk of tracheal and stomal inflammation, infection, and mucous plugs

ARTIFICIAL AIRWAYS CONTINUED

AIRWAY INSERTION TIPS

An unconscious patient may need an oropharyngeal airway to prevent his tongue from slipping back and blocking his pharynx. He may need a nasopharyngeal airway if he's conscious, needs frequent nasotracheal suctioning, or has facial injuries that contraindicate an oral airway. Review the following points for insertion technique guidelines. But remember, the patient's natural airway *must be unobstructed* before you attempt to insert any type of artificial airway. *Note:* If your patient's wearing dentures, remove them first.

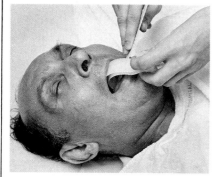

To insert an oropharyngeal airway:
• The quickest way to insert this airway is by pointing its tip toward the roof of the mouth. Gently advance the airway by rotating it 180°. If the patient gags during insertion, pause and wait for him to stop; then proceed.
• Here's an alternate method: Hold down the patient's tongue with a tongue depressor and guide the airway over the back of his tongue until it's in position. (This technique works well with infants.)
• When the airway's in place, position the patient's head to one side to decrease the risk of aspiration if he vomits. Then tape the top and bottom of the airway to his cheeks. (Take care to leave enough room for suctioning.)

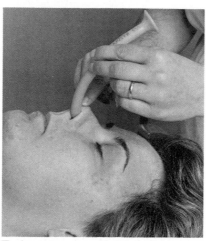

To insert a nasopharyngeal airway:
• Use a tube with an outside diameter that's slightly larger than the patient's nostril.
• Then determine the correct tube length for the patient by measuring from the tip of his nose to to his earlobe. Mark the distance on the tube; you'll insert the tube to this depth.
• Lubricate the tube with water or water-soluble jelly. Reassure the patient and explain what you're going to do. Position him flat on his back and push up the tip of his nose. Insert the tube up to the mark you've made.
• To check for proper positioning, ask him to exhale with his mouth closed. You should feel air leaving the tube. Also check visually, by holding the patient's mouth open with a tongue depressor and looking for the tube's tip just behind the uvula.

YOUR ROLE IN EMERGENCY TRACHEOTOMY

Under ordinary circumstances, the doctor would perform a tracheotomy only in the operating room. But in an emergency, when every second counts, he may perform the procedure at the patient's bedside. Indications for such a step include airway obstruction by laryngeal edema and failure of other methods to open the airway.

Preparation. To assist with the procedure, first gather the necessary equipment: trach tray, sterile gloves, antimicrobial solution (such as povidone-iodine) sterile water, 3-0 and 4-0 size silk sutures, 22G needle, 5-ml syringe, a local anesthetic, and suctioning equipment (including gloves and sterile saline solution). Then position the patient flat on his back, and place a small rolled towel under his shoulder blades to hyperextend his neck and properly align his trachea. If he's conscious, explain what's happening and offer reassurance. *Note:* If time permits, make sure an appropriate person has signed a consent form, according to hospital policy.

Remove the headboard of the bed so you can easily position yourself to provide artificial ventilation if necessary. Make sure the bedside area is well lighted.

Surgery. To make the incision, the doctor will first split the patient's thyroid gland and hold it back with retractors. Then he'll make an incision in the trachea below the cricoid cartilage.

After the doctor's inserted the trach tube and completed the procedure, document it in your nurse's notes. Observe the patient closely for signs of bleeding or edema, and notify the doctor immediately if either develops.

ESOPHAGEAL AIRWAYS: STOPGAP EMERGENCY MEASURES

In a respiratory crisis occurring outside the hospital, such specially trained personnel as emergency medical technicians may have to insert an esophageal gastric tube airway (EGTA) (see photo) or an esophageal obturator airway (EOA) in the patient. The EGTA is used for patients who need a nasogastric tube, since it has a port for tube insertion.

These temporary devices can help emergency medical personnel ventilate an unconscious patient, until he reaches the hospital, by:
• preventing tongue obstruction
• preventing air from entering the stomach
• blocking stomach contents from entering the trachea.

The EGTA and EOA are contraindicated in patients under age 16, since pediatric sizes aren't currently available. They should also be avoided in a patient who lacks a strong gag reflex or who's ingested a toxic chemical.

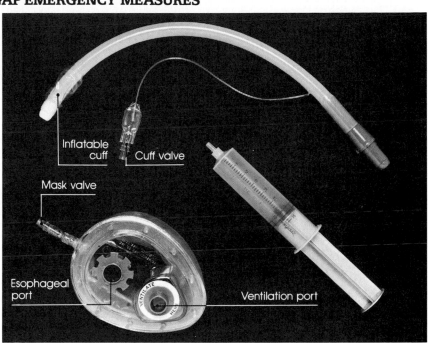

CRICOID STAB: A LAST RESORT

At the scene of an accident or an emergency outside the hospital, you may have no alternative but to perform a cricoid stab (emergency cricothyreotomy) to open someone's airway. In such an extreme emergency, when all else fails, follow these steps:
• Gently grasp the patient's trachea. Slide your fingers downward to find his thyroid gland. You've located its outer borders when the space between your fingers and thumb widens.
• Move your index finger across the center of the gland over the anterior edge of the cricoid ring.
• Cut or stab the patient's cricothyroid membrane, just below the cricoid ring, using scissors or a pocket knife. Insert something hollow—for example, a drinking straw or plastic pen with ink cartridge removed—to keep the airway open.

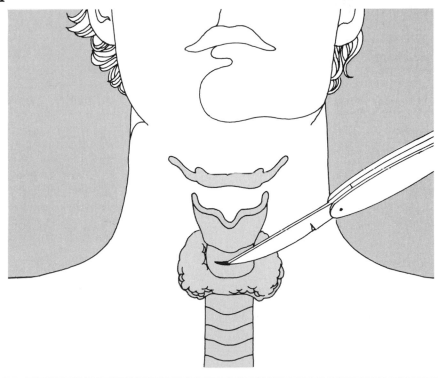

ARTIFICIAL AIRWAYS CONTINUED

COMMON TUBE PROBLEMS

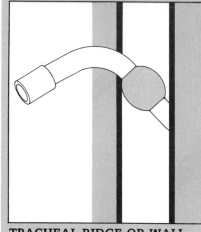 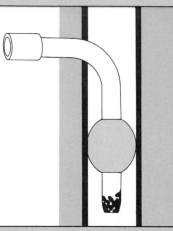 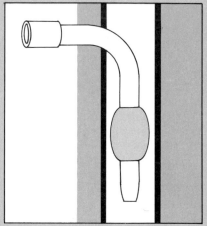

TRACHEAL RIDGE OR WALL OBSTRUCTS TUBE LUMEN

Signs
• Difficulty in forcing air into the tube with a hand-held ventilator
• Obstruction in the tube during suctioning
• Decrease in PaO_2 indicated by patient's blood gas values
• Activation of ventilator's pressure alarm
• Patient anxious and agitated (air hunger)

Treatment
• Deflate cuff and reposition tube.
• Secure the tube with tape.

Prevention
• Make sure the proper size tube has been selected.
• Tape the tube securely.
• Tie the trach ties snugly.

SECRETIONS OBSTRUCT TUBE LUMEN

Signs
• Obstruction in the tube when suctioning
• Decrease in PaO_2 indicated by patient's blood gas values
• Activation of ventilator's pressure alarm

Treatment
• Move suction catheter to one side to bypass obstruction.
• Instill saline solution, hyperinflate the patient's lungs, and suction him with the correct size catheter.
• Humidify the patient's airway.
• Perform postural drainage, percussion, and vibration.
• If ordered, change the tube.

Prevention
• As ordered, use humidified oxygen to keep secretions thin.
• If ordered, perform periodic cooled or heated aerosol treatments.
• Exercise meticulous trach care.
• If ordered, administer forced fluids or I.V. therapy.

UNDERINFLATED CUFF

Signs
• Significant air leak through the patient's stoma, nose, or mouth
• Decrease in expired air volume, indicated by spirometer reading on ventilator

Treatment
• Inflate cuff to the proper size, using the minimal air-leak technique. (See page 56.)

Prevention
• Follow the manufacturer's recommendations on cuff volume as an initial guide for inflation. But, also use the minimal air-leak technique.
• Measure cuff pressure immediately after inflation and routinely check pressure.

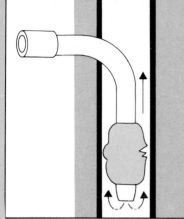

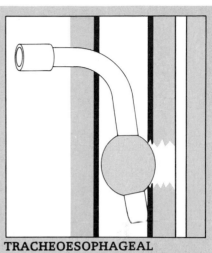

RUPTURED CUFF
Signs
• Significant air leak through the patient's stoma, nose, or mouth
• No pressure registered on manometer check
• Decrease in expired air volume, indicated by spirometer reading on ventilator
• Activation of ventilator's low-pressure alarm
• Patient can talk
Treatment
• Notify the doctor. He may order the tube changed.
Prevention
• Check the cuff for symmetrical inflation before the tube is inserted.
• Avoid accidentally pulling the cuff into the suction catheter when performing nasotracheal suctioning.

HERNIATED CUFF BLOCKING END OF TUBE
Signs
• Obstruction in the tube during suctioning
• Decrease in PaO_2 indicated by patient's blood gas values
• Activation of ventilator's low-pressure alarm
• Moderate difficulty on inhalation; exhalation may be completely blocked
Treatment
• Replace the trach tube immediately.
• Keep an extra tube on hand in case the doctor orders a replacement.
Prevention
• Check the cuff for symmetrical inflation before tube insertion.
• Avoid overinflating the cuff.

TRACHEOESOPHAGEAL FISTULA
Signs
• Significant air leak through the patient's stoma, nose, or mouth, even though cuff is adequately inflated
• Food or liquid present in the aspirate during suctioning
• Frequent belching
• Coughing with each attempt to swallow
• Positive methylene blue test results, if your patient can swallow (Ask him to drink methylene blue or another dark liquid. Then suction the tube. If a fistula's present, tracheal secretions will be stained dark.)
Treatment
• Don't feed the patient until extent of fistula is determined.
• Suction his trachea through the tube only.
• If ordered, remove the endotracheal tube.
• If ordered, administer total parenteral nutrition.
Prevention
• Use a low-pressure cuff.
• Use minimal air-leak technique to inflate cuff.
• Exercise meticulous cuff care.
• Don't leave an oral endotracheal tube in place for extended periods of time.

ARTIFICIAL AIRWAYS CONTINUED

MINIMAL AIR-LEAK TECHNIQUE

Underinflating a trach tube cuff causes air leaks around the cuff; overinflating can cause cuff rupture or tracheal damage. Avoid these problems by using the minimal air-leak technique, as shown at right:

• Suction the patient's oropharynx and trachea.
• Insert a syringe into the valve at the end of the cuff pillow. Deflate the cuff by aspirating air until you feel resistance. Then, draw back on the plunger slightly. Press the pillow repeatedly.
• Now, inflate the cuff during inspiration. Place your stethoscope on one side of the patient's trachea and listen for gurgling or squeaking sounds, which indicate a leak.
• If no leak is present, slowly remove 0.2 to 0.3 cc more air, and listen again for gurgling or squeaking sounds.
• If all's well, check the cuff pressure; it should be less than 15 mm Hg or 25 cmH$_2$O. If cuff pressure is higher—or if you detected a leak—prepare to replace the defective trach tube.
• To avoid overinflation, measure cuff pressure every 8 hours.

Make sure the patient's in the same position each time you measure. (A position change can alter the pressure needed to achieve an adequate seal.)

SUCTIONING GUIDELINES

A patient with an artificial airway needs regular suctioning. To do this safely and effectively, follow these rules:

• Explain the procedure to your patient, emphasizing that suctioning will help him breathe more easily.
• If possible, help him deep breathe and cough before suctioning.
• If he's receiving continuous oxygen therapy, hyperventilate his lungs for several minutes before and after suctioning. Reset the oxygen flow rate after hyperventilation.
• Never suction for longer than 12 seconds. If necessary, encourage the patient to breathe deeply for at least 1 minute; then repeat the procedure.
• If his secretions are tenacious, place the catheter tip in the saline solution and apply suction to clear it.
• After suctioning, immediately reconnect the patient to the ventilator or oxygen-delivery system.

Don't rush the procedure. Your patient will be more relaxed if you take your time.

• Discard the used suction catheter, gloves, and basin; make sure new equipment is available at the bedside.
• Wrap the connector tube around the suction gauge to keep it out of the way.
• Auscultate the patient's lungs bilaterally to assess the procedure's effectiveness. Both fields should be clear.
• Complete mouth care, as indicated.
• Document the procedure, including the amount, color, and consistency of suctioned secretions.
• Replace saline solution and sterile water with a fresh supply every 24 hours. Write the date and time you opened each bottle on the labels.
• Empty and rinse vacuum bottles at the end of each shift or more frequently, if necessary. Never allow contents to fill above overflow line.

SPECIAL PROBLEMS

NURSING CHECKLIST

ANAPHYLAXIS

You can't always anticipate whom anaphylaxis will strike—or how quickly. This life-threatening systemic reaction sometimes develops unexpectedly in patients who have no history of allergy. In some cases, signs and symptoms appear within seconds of exposure to the allergen; in others, up to 1 hour later. But regardless of the circumstances, an untreated patient can die quickly from airway obstruction (caused by laryngeal edema) and shock.

The faster a patient's symptoms develop, the more likely the reaction will be fatal. To save an anaphylactic patient, immediately take these steps:

• Make sure he has an open airway. Prepare to assist with endotracheal tube insertion or an emergency tracheotomy, if necessary. Keep in mind that an artificial oral airway won't keep the airway open if extreme laryngeal edema develops.

• Administer epinephrine to block the release of histamine and counteract histamine's effects (for example, bronchospasm and vasodilation). If your patient has an I.V. in place, give 0.1 to 0.25 ml 1:1,000 I.V. Or, give 0.3 to 0.5 ml 1:1,000 subcutaneously. Increase the dose to 1 ml for intramuscular injection. Repeat the dose every 10 minutes, as ordered, until the patient's out of danger.

• Give corticosteroids I.V. or antihistamines I.M. if ordered.

• If symptoms persist, start an I.V. with lactated Ringer's solution, using a large-bore catheter. Fluid administration helps counteract the hypovolemia associated with shock.

• If epinephrine fails to control the patient's anaphylaxis, give a vasopressor, such as norepinephrine (Levophed), as ordered: 8 to 12 mcg/minute initially, then 2 to 4 mcg/minute. Closely monitor blood pressure and watch the infusion site for signs of infiltration. *Note:* Depending on the reaction's severity, the doctor may also order dopamine (Intropin) to maintain blood pressure and prevent further systemic reactions, and aminophylline to combat bronchospasms.

• Closely monitor the patient's vital signs throughout treatment and recovery. Watch particularly for adverse reactions to emergency drugs; for example, tachycardia from epinephrine or dizziness from the antihistamine.

• Teach the patient how to avoid future episodes. Advise him to wear a Medic Alert tag and to inform all health-care professionals who treat him of his allergy.

ACUTE EPIGLOTTITIS: THE CHILD KILLER

Rare in adults, acute epiglottitis most often strikes children between ages 2 and 12. Because this bacterial infection causes inflammation and edema of the epiglottis, 8% to 12% of its victims suffocate before anyone can help them.

Assessment. Because complete airway obstruction can develop in 2 to 5 hours, your prompt recognition of impending obstruction is critical. Look for these danger signs: history of recent upper respiratory infection; high fever; sore throat; dysphagia; stridor on inspiration; severe dyspnea; nostril flaring; muffled voice sounds; drooling; irritability or restlessness; rhonchi; and inspiratory retractions.

To relieve his breathing difficulty, the child may sit upright or lean forward with his neck hyperextended and his tongue protruding—a pose characteristic of epiglottitis.

Intervention. Immediately report the above danger signs to the doctor and make sure emergency equipment, including a tracheotomy tray, is on hand.

After the doctor's diagnosed the problem, prepare the child for transfer to the intensive care unit. Explain the child's condition and treatment to his parents, and prepare them for the possibility of an emergency tracheotomy or endotracheal intubation.

Special Note:

If you suspect epiglottitis, don't use a tongue depressor to examine the child's throat. Doing so can trigger sudden and complete airway obstruction.

C.O.P.D. BASICS

C.O.P.D.: BRONCHIAL AIRWAY OBSTRUCTION

Unlike upper airway obstructions, which are usually acute conditions, lower airway obstructions are chronic and progressive conditions punctuated by acute episodes. Commonly grouped under the umbrella term *chronic obstructive pulmonary disease* (COPD), these conditions include bronchitis, emphysema, and asthma. Although each condition has a distinctive pathophysiology, all are characterized by a narrowing of bronchial airways. By trapping air in the bronchioles and alveoli, this narrowing impairs ventilation, hinders gas exchange, and distends the alveoli.

Who's at risk. What causes COPD? The most important single predisposing factor is cigarette smoking; COPD is relatively rare in nonsmokers. Habitual smoking impairs ciliary action and macrophagic activity, causes airway inflammation and excessive mucus production, destroys alveolar septae, and encourages the development of peribronchiolar fibrosis. Prolonged exposure to irritating dust, fibers, and fumes—especially in combination with cigarette smoking—produces similar effects.

Other significant risk factors include the following:

• *Hereditary predisposition* contributes significantly to the development of asthma and—in some patients—emphysema. For example, an inherited deficiency of alpha$_1$-antitrypsin, a nonspecific proteolytic enzyme inhibitor, permits naturally occurring proteolytic enzymes to cause lung tissue lysis; this, in turn, leads to emphysema.

• *Aging* may be associated with mild panlobular emphysema, an often asymptomatic condition common among elderly patients.

• *Respiratory infection* is the primary cause of intrinsic (nonatopic) asthma. In addition, infections exacerbate all COPD types.

C.O.P.D. deaths

Deaths from COPD and related conditions totaled over 64,000 in 1983.

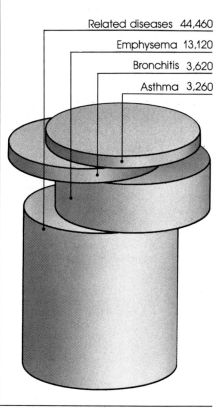

Related diseases 44,460
Emphysema 13,120
Bronchitis 3,620
Asthma 3,260

C.O.P.D. COMPLICATIONS

The COPD patient's predisposed to several serious complications that could lead to death. By understanding how these complications arise and doing your best to prevent them, you *can* make a difference. Significant complications include:

• *Infection.* The COPD patient's highly susceptible to lung-damaging infection, which can set the stage for reinfection, respiratory irritation, or a potential allergic reaction.

What makes the COPD patient so vulnerable? He usually produces excessive mucus that becomes trapped along with air and bacteria in the tracheobronchial tract. COPD also impairs effective coughing and deep exhalations—important cleansing mechanisms.

As a result, protective cilia are destroyed.

And because the COPD patient breathes through his mouth, his secretions become dry and difficult to expel. The result: buildup of mucus, the perfect medium for bacterial growth.

• *Pulmonary hypertension.* Because lung congestion reduces the space of the pulmonary vascular bed, pulmonary arterial pressure rises, possibly causing pulmonary hypertension.

Polycythemia, a response to the COPD patient's hypoxia, contributes to pulmonary hypertension by increasing blood viscosity, which distends blood vessels and makes the heart work harder. In some cases, pulmonary hypertension brings on cor pul-

monale—right ventricular hypertrophy.

• *Right heart failure.* In advanced COPD, peripheral edema and venous distention can cause right heart failure—a potentially fatal development.

• *Acute respiratory failure.* Emphysema—particularly the advanced stage—may severely impair the brain's respiratory center, reducing cerebral oxygenation, increasing $PaCO_2$ levels, and possibly causing hypoxia and respiratory acidosis. If respiratory impairment continues, the patient may die.

• *Status asthmaticus.* This acute, prolonged attack may develop if standard asthma medication doesn't relieve bronchospasm.

ANALYZING AN ASTHMA ATTACK

Asthma is characterized by spasms of bronchial (and bronchiolar) smooth muscle that narrow lower airway passages and cause diffuse airway obstruction.

What causes an asthma attack? No one knows exactly; however, an attack may be associated with one or more of the following: allergy, infection, exposure to respiratory irritants, and emotional or psychological distress. Asthma's commonly classified as *intrinsic* or *extrinsic*. We'll explain these two types in detail on the next page.

During a typical asthma attack, an inflammatory response encourages airway obstruction by engorging blood vessels and swelling mucous glands and goblet cells. This, in turn, increases mucus production and compounds the problem.

As in emphysema, expiration is more difficult than inspiration; this accounts for the prolonged expiration time and wheezing that accompany an asthma attack. If the attack worsens, hyperinflation of the distal airways increases—the result of premature airway closure, mucous plugs, edema, and increased expiration time (from increased airway resistance). As the lungs absorb trapped air, areas of atelectasis may develop.

Meanwhile, the patient's growing anxiety increases his body's metabolic demands. The lungs, hampered by defective gas exchange, can't meet the increased demand, thus causing hypoxia. The patient also experiences fatigue, systolic hypertension, diaphoresis, coughing, and possibly mental confusion and asterixis (flapping tremor).

A prolonged asthma attack that doesn't respond to bronchodilators and other routine therapy is a medical emergency called *status asthmaticus*. Most asthma attacks, however, are short-lived and reversible. Some patients have prolonged, symptom-free periods between attacks. But chronic, sustained attacks can cause smooth muscle hypertrophy and permanent narrowing of the respiratory tract.

How asthma obstructs the bronchial airways

As this illustration shows, asthma narrows the bronchioles. Compare the normal bronchiole (top close-up) with the obstructed bronchiole (bottom close-up). In response to smooth muscle spasms and inflammation, the affected bronchiole fills with engorged blood vessels, swollen mucous glands, goblet cells, and mucous secretions containing various substances.

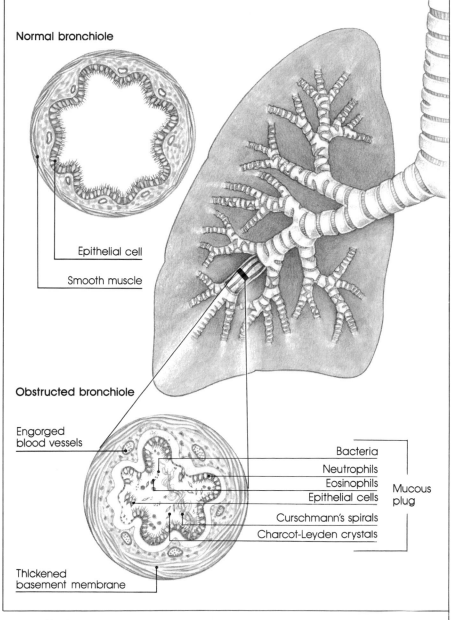

Normal bronchiole

Epithelial cell

Smooth muscle

Obstructed bronchiole

Engorged blood vessels

Bacteria
Neutrophils
Eosinophils
Epithelial cells

Mucous plug

Curschmann's spirals
Charcot-Leyden crystals

Thickened basement membrane

C.O.P.D. BASICS CONTINUED

IDENTIFYING ASTHMA TYPES

To classify your patient's asthma, consider which factors precipitate his attacks.

• *Extrinsic* (allergic) asthma is triggered by an allergic reaction to dust, pollen, animal dander, or other allergens. Typically, patients prone to this asthma type have high serum levels of immunoglobulin E (IgE) antibodies, produced in response to exposure to the offending allergen. These antibodies attach to mast cells in the submucosa of bronchial epithelium, where they trigger an antigen-antibody reaction in response to subsequent allergen exposure.

A complete medical history can help identify the cause of a patient's extrinsic asthma.

Extrinsic asthma's most common among young asthmatic patients with a history of infantile eczema or allergic rhinitis. The doctor diagnoses the condition from a serum analysis that reveals IgE antibodies. To determine allergic response to specific antigens, he'll order skin tests.

• *Intrinsic* (nonallergic or perennial) asthma's more common among older patients. Apparently unrelated to allergic reactions, intrinsic asthma attacks may be associated with respiratory tract infections, exercise, cold air, smoke and other pollutants, or emotional distress.

• *Mixed asthma* stems from both allergic and nonallergic factors.

BRONCHITIS: AIRWAY INFLAMMATION

Marked by inflammation of the distal airways, bronchitis usually develops after long-term exposure to cigarette smoke or air pollution. Tissue irritation causes vasodilation, congestion, mucosal edema, and hypertrophy of mucus-secreting goblet cells, which then copiously produce mucus. At the same time, tissue inflammation reduces the number and efficiency of cilia lining the airway, decreasing the respiratory tract's ability to clear mucous secretions. As a result, the patient develops a productive cough—commonly called cigarette cough or smoker's hack—that's worse during the morning. This chronic cough contributes to progressive destruction of smaller bronchioles, perpetuating the patient's symptoms.

As the condition progresses, increasingly thick, tenacious mucous secretions obstruct the airway, causing inadequate gas exchange and dyspnea on exertion. Fewer alveoli are fully ventilated, causing first a decreased PaO_2 level, then an elevated $PaCO_2$ level.

But even when the patient becomes hypoxic and hypercapnic, he probably won't develop compensatory hyperventilation. The reason is that the brain's respiratory center and central chemoreceptors, which normally correct arterial blood gas imbalances by increasing the respiratory rate, become increasingly insensitive to sustained hypercapnia.

Secondary to low PaO_2 levels, pulmonary vasoconstriction may occur, increasing pulmonary vascular pressure. Because this additional pressure increases resistance to right ventricular outflow, the right ventricle must work harder. In time, its increased work load may cause right ventricular hypertrophy and failure, with edema.

How bronchitis alters bronchiolar tissue

In the bronchiole illustrated below, the left portion shows healthy tissue with normal mucous glands. In acute bronchitis, inflammation causes mucous glands to increase in size and number, as shown on the right.

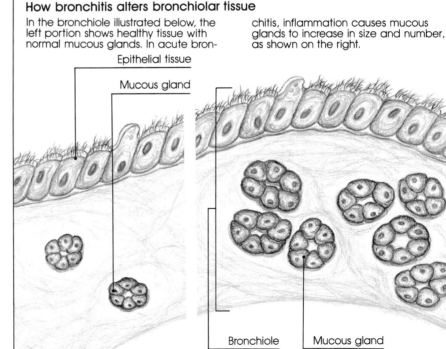

Epithelial tissue

Mucous gland

Bronchiole   Mucous gland

EMPHYSEMA: A SURPLUS OF ALVEOLAR AIR

Although emphysema sometimes occurs by itself, it more commonly develops after a long history of chronic bronchitis; indeed, this disease combination is the classic COPD. Despite this relationship, however, emphysema differs significantly—in both pathophysiology and symptoms—from bronchitis. While bronchitis limits both inhalation and exhalation, emphysema primarily restricts exhalation.

Normally, exhalation is passive, powered by the elastic recoil of healthy lung tissue. Emphysema causes anatomic changes in the lung that destroy its elasticity. As a result, the patient begins to have difficulty exhaling.

Why does emphysema often succeed long-standing bronchitis?

The increased mucus production that accompanies bronchitis blocks the small terminal bronchioles, trapping air in the alveoli. Recurrent inflammation, associated with the release of proteolytic enzymes from lung cells, contributes to the breakdown of alveolar walls, bronchioles, and connective tissue. Clusters of alveoli merge, reducing the number of alveoli and increasing the number of air spaces available to trap inhaled air. The combination of trapped air and alveolar distention eventually causes the patient to develop a barrel chest—a round, bulging chest with increased anteroposterior diameter.

Alveolar wall destruction also causes the small airways to col-

lapse during exhalation and disrupts the lungs' capillary bed, reducing lung tissue perfusion. However, alveolar and vascular changes vary throughout the lung. Some areas become overventilated in relation to tissue perfusion; others are underventilated.

Because overventilated areas usually predominate, the patient will probably maintain relatively normal oxygen saturation and thus escape the cyanosis that may plague a bronchitis sufferer. But the patient with emphysema may eventually develop hypercapnia and respiratory acidosis. If the condition progresses, the brain's respiratory control centers become desensitized to hypercapnia. Hypoxemia then becomes the stimulus for breathing.

CLASSIFYING EMPHYSEMA

Depending on the specific anatomic changes your patient has experienced, classify emphysema as follows:
• *Centrilobular* emphysema, the most common type, often occurs with chronic bronchitis. Bronchioles in the lungs' upper or central portions enlarge and merge, impairing gas diffusion.
• *Panlobular* emphysema, which affects the lungs' basal portions, systematically destroys and dilates air spaces distal to the terminal bronchioles. All air spaces are affected uniformly, and surrounding tissue deteriorates. Characterized by diminished alveolar-capillary surface area, panlobular emphysema is often associated with alpha$_1$-antitrypsin deficiency.
• *Paraseptal* emphysema results from any condition causing scarring or fibrosis. It's characterized by alveolar wall destruction, alveolar distention adjacent to fibrotic lesions, and focal air cysts.

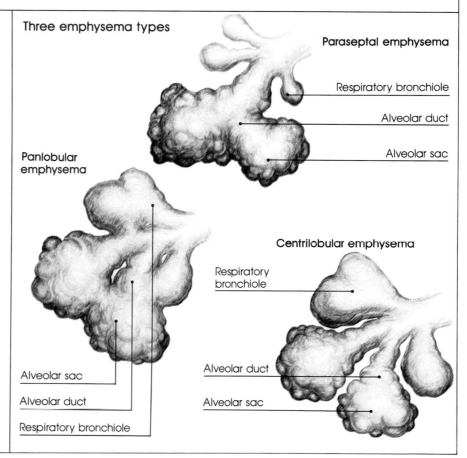

Three emphysema types

Paraseptal emphysema

Respiratory bronchiole

Alveolar duct

Alveolar sac

Panlobular emphysema

Centrilobular emphysema

Respiratory bronchiole

Alveolar duct

Alveolar sac

Alveolar sac

Alveolar duct

Respiratory bronchiole

C.O.P.D. ASSESSMENT

C.O.P.D. ASSESSMENT FINDINGS

Use this chart to compare the three primary causes of COPD. But remember, assessment findings may vary from one patient to the next, depending on the condition's severity and the presence or absence of complications.

CHRONIC BRONCHITIS

Onset

Insidious; usually affects patients over age 40 who smoke

Signs and symptoms
• Chronic, productive cough that's worse in the mornings and during cold weather
• Exertional dyspnea
• Use of accessory muscles for breathing
• Rhonchi and wheezes on auscultation

History
• Long-term smoking
• Chronic cough for at least 3 months a year for two successive years
• Recurrent episodes of diaphoresis (especially at night)
• Recurrent respiratory tract infections

Diagnostic test results
• *Chest X-ray:* may show hyperinflation and increased bronchovascular markings
• *Pulmonary function tests:* normal in early stage; as condition progresses, tests show increased residual volume, decreased vital capacity and forced expiratory volumes, normal static compliance and diffusing capacity
• *Arterial blood gases (ABGs):* decreased PaO_2, normal or elevated $PaCO_2$
• *Sputum:* thick; grey, yellow, or white; contains microorganisms and neutrophils
• *EKG:* may show atrial dysrhythmias; peaked P waves in leads II, III, and aVF; and possibly right ventricular hypertrophy
• *Complete blood count:* elevated leukocytes if a bacterial infection's present

EMPHYSEMA

Onset

Insidious; most often affects patients over age 60

Signs and symptoms
• Exertional dyspnea
• Chronic but relatively unproductive cough
• Weight loss, prolonged expiratory period with grunting, pursed-lip breathing, tachypnea
• Use of accessory muscles to breathe
• Hyperresonance on percussion, increased breath sounds, quiet heart sounds
• Anorexia and malaise
• Barrel chest
• Peripheral cyanosis and digital clubbing

History
• Chronic cough and exertional dyspnea for 5 years or more
• Long-term smoker and/or history of bronchitis
• Recurrent respiratory tract infections
• Family history of asthma or alpha$_1$-antitrypsin deficiency

Diagnostic test results
• *Chest X-ray:* in moderate to advanced disease, flattened diaphragm, reduced vascular markings at lung periphery, over-aeration of lungs, vertical heart, enlarged anteroposterior chest diameter, large retrosternal air space
• *Pulmonary function tests:* in moderate to advanced disease, increased total lung capacity and residual volume, decreased vital capacity and forced expiratory volumes, increased static compliance and decreased expiratory volumes
• *ABGs:* reduced PaO_2; normal $PaCO_2$ (until late in the disease)
• *EKG:* tall, symmetric P waves in leads II, III, and aVF; vertical QRS axis, signs of right ventricular hypertrophy late in disease
• *Complete blood count:* increased hemoglobin late in disease when persistent severe hypoxia develops

ASTHMA

Onset

Childhood onset associated with allergy; adult onset may be unrelated to allergy

Signs and symptoms
During an attack:
• Mild to severe dyspnea and wheezing
• Chest tightness
• Productive cough (clear, white, or yellow tenacious mucus)
• Hyperinflated chest
• Flared nostrils
• Anxiety
• Use of accessory muscles to breathe
• Diaphoresis
• Tachycardia, hypertension, pulsus paradoxus
• On auscultation, rhonchi and wheezing throughout lung fields on expiration and possibly inspiration; absent or diminished breath sounds during severe obstruction. Unequal intensity of breath sounds reflects uneven air distribution in the lungs. Bilateral wheezing may be audible without a stethoscope. *Note:* In severe airway obstruction, wheezing and rhonchi diminish or disappear.

Between attacks:
• Patient may be asymptomatic
• Chronic sustained attacks may

C.O.P.D. MANAGEMENT

lead to smooth muscle hypertrophy and may narrow the respiratory tract; patient may then develop chronic symptoms similar to those caused by chronic bronchitis and emphysema

History
• Intermittent attacks of dyspnea and wheezing; may occur most often at night, after exposure to certain allergens, or during periods of emotional stress
• Eczema, urticaria, seasonal or other allergies (including allergies to aspirin or other drugs), sinus problems, colds and other respiratory infections, or nasal polyps

Diagnostic tests results
During an attack:
• *Chest X-ray:* hyperinflated lungs with air trapping; areas of atelectasis possible
• *Sputum:* presence of Curschmann's spirals (airway casts), eosinophils, and Charcot-Leyden crystals (breakdown products from eosinophils)
• *Pulmonary function tests:* decreased forced expiratory volume that improves significantly after administration of inhalation bronchodilator; increased residual volume and functional residual capacity; total lung capacity may also increase
• *ABGs:* decreased PaO_2; $PaCO_2$ values variable. *Caution:* Rising $PaCO_2$ levels and decreasing pH indicate acidosis and impending respiratory failure
• *EKG:* sinus tachycardia; during severe attack, signs of cor pulmonale (right axis deviation, peaked P wave) may appear

SETTING GOALS
In any respiratory disorder, your goal is to maintain a patent airway. To achieve that goal in a patient with acute asthma, bronchitis, or emphysema, take immediate steps to:
• relieve bronchospasm
• reduce mucosal edema
• improve expectoration.

In most cases, drugs and physiotherapy (discussed in detail on the next few pages) can help the patient achieve his baseline pulmonary function. (Since COPD is chronic and progressive, it's unrealistic to try to reestablish normal pulmonary function.)

Drug therapy for COPD consists primarily of oral bronchodilators (to open obstructed airways) and parenteral administration of adrenergic drugs (to produce bronchodilation and facilitate mucus transport) and steroids (to reduce bronchial edema and inflammation). Chest physiotherapy can help loosen and remove mucus from the tracheobronchial tree.

Your patient will need special care throughout his treatment to prevent such complications as infection, pulmonary hypertension, and cardiac or respiratory failure. By carefully monitoring his status, paying close attention to even the slightest change, you can help protect him from these potentially life-threatening developments.

But the COPD patient needs more than just appropriate medical intervention to relieve his physical distress. He also needs emotional support. As he fights what may seem like a losing battle to get enough air, he may become anxious, as well as physically exhausted. Hypoxia and hypercapnia, which accompany acute COPD episodes, may make him confused, and such drugs as aminophylline and theophylline given to relieve his symptoms may cause restlessness. He may also complain of dizziness and insomnia. To help minimize his emotional distress, reassure him frequently that the episode will pass. If you must leave his room, tell him where you're going and when you'll be back.

Once the crisis is over, tell the patient that he can reduce the frequency and severity of future acute episodes by avoiding bronchopulmonary irritants, particularly cigarette smoke, and contact with respiratory infections. Effective coughing and deep breathing techniques may also help, particularly for a patient with bronchitis or emphysema.

On the next few pages, we'll take a closer look at emergency care for patients in acute stages of COPD, as well as self-care methods that can prevent recurring episodes.

Special Note:
Never administer a high percentage of oxygen to a patient with chronic asthma or another form of COPD. If you do, he may stop breathing. Here's why: A normal person breathes because his respiratory system's stimulated by an increased $PaCO_2$ level. But a COPD patient may consistently retain a high level of carbon dioxide from hypoventilation. Over time, his respiratory center compensates, no longer responding to increased $PaCO_2$ levels. Hypoxia then becomes his only breathing stimulus. Administering oxygen at a high percentage would depress his hypoxic drive and lead to respiratory arrest.

C.O.P.D. MANAGEMENT CONTINUED

EMPHYSEMA AND BRONCHITIS: CARE PRIORITIES

When exacerbated by a concurrent illness, chronic bronchitis or emphysema can become a medical emergency. Because these two diseases are so closely linked, emergency treatment is basically the same.

The patient with acute bronchitis or emphysema will be struggling frantically for air. Your first priority is to position him in a way that will relieve his respiratory distress. For most patients, a high Fowler's position allows maximum diaphragmatic expansion and decreases air trapping. Other patients may be helped by sitting on the edge of the bed and leaning forward across a pillow placed on an overbed table. Remember to reassure the patient.

Treatment of acute bronchitis or emphysema usually involves the following:
• oxygen at 2 liters/minute
• I.V. infusion of dextrose 5% in water
• a bronchodilator, such as aminophylline, administered via continuous I.V. infusion
• corticosteroids, such as beclomethasone, administered via aerosol therapy, or methylprednisolone administered I.V.
• antibiotics (usually ampicillin or tetracycline) and expectorants, if an infection's suspected
• adequate hydration. To help remove mucous plugs and counteract dehydration, the patient with acute bronchitis may require up to 4 liters of fluid daily by mouth. A patient with acute emphysema requires less fluid since mucus buildup from emphysema is usually minimal.
• chest physiotherapy, specifically percussion and postural drainage. (For details, see the photostory on the opposite page.)

NEBULIZER THERAPY: ENSURING PROPER TECHNIQUE

The goal of nebulizer therapy is to deliver an adequate concentration of medication to receptor sites deep in the patient's airways. Improper nebulizer use could decrease the concentration below therapeutic levels or increase it to toxic levels. To ensure that your patient with acute COPD receives maximum benefits from nebulizer therapy, make sure he's using the nebulizer correctly. Review these techniques:
• So the medication will deeply penetrate the airways, instruct the patient to hold the nebulizer about 2" from his open mouth, with his head tilted back slightly.

Note: Advise him to inspect the nebulizer carefully before each use to make sure no foreign objects (for example, small coins, buttons, or pins) have become lodged in the mouthpiece. Also teach him how to store the nebulizer properly between uses. In one reported incident, a patient inhaled a dime that had found its way into his fully assembled nebulizer, which had been in his pocket.
• Next, the patient should exhale normally, then inhale deeply and slowly for about 5 seconds while depressing the top of the nebulizer's metal canister. Deep, slow inhalation allows more medication to reach the small airways and helps the lungs retain the medication.
• To prevent the patient from exhaling medication that would otherwise reach his lungs, tell him to hold his breath for 3 to 5 seconds after inhaling. If a second inhalation is needed, he should allow 5 to 10 minutes for the first dose to take effect before repeating the procedure.

Note: If the patient's receiving both a bronchodilator (such as metaproterenol) and a corticosteroid (such as beclomethasone), administer the bronchodilator first. This dilates the airways, allowing the corticosteroid to be inhaled more deeply.

How to use a hand-held nebulizer

To permit nebulizer medication to fully penetrate the lungs (as in the illustration below), the patient must inhale slowly and deeply, then hold his breath for 3 to 5 seconds.

If the patient inhales for only 1 or 2 seconds, the medication may not reach the small airways (see illustration below).

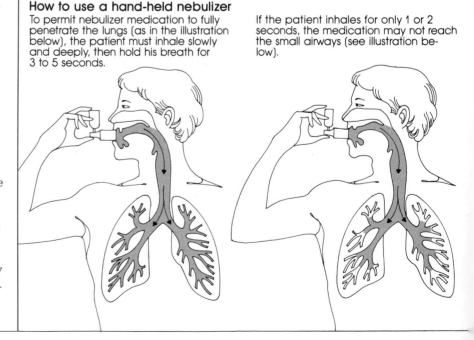

PERFORMING CHEST PHYSIOTHERAPY

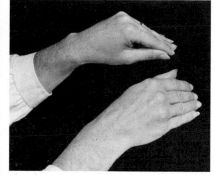

1 To relieve a COPD patient's lung congestion, the doctor may order chest physiotherapy, such as percussion and postural drainage. By mobilizing secretions, these techniques help clear the airways and improve ventilation. To percuss, hold your hands in a cupped shape. Keep your hands flexed and your thumbs tight against your index fingers. As you alternate your hands rhythmically, try to trap air between your hands and the patient's chest.

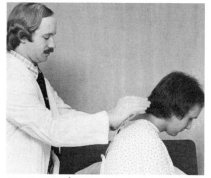

2 To drain the apical segments of both upper lung lobes, seat your patient on the edge of his bed and support his feet. Then ask him to tip his head forward slightly. Standing behind him, percuss his upper back and shoulders as close as possible to the apex of his shoulder blades.

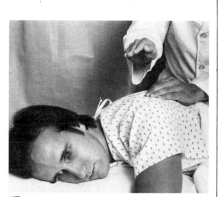

3 To drain the posterior segment of his left upper lobe, raise the head of the bed slightly. Position your patient so he's lying partly on his right side and partly on his abdomen, hugging a pillow as shown here. Use both hands to percuss the patient's back, near his left scapula. Don't percuss over the bony shoulder blade.

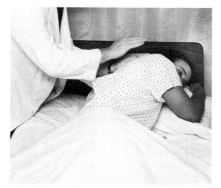

4 To drain the posterior segment of the right upper lobe, lower the bed until it's flat. Position your patient so he's lying partly on his left side and partly on his abdomen, hugging a pillow. Then, percuss his back near his right scapula, as shown here.

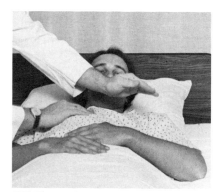

5 To drain the anterior portions of both upper lobes, keep the bed flat. Position your patient on his back. Then, percuss both sides of his upper chest below the clavicle.

When you percuss a woman, work *around* her breasts, not *over* them, to avoid causing pain. If her breasts are too large to percuss around, use an alternate method; for example, postural drainage by itself or with mechanical percussor.

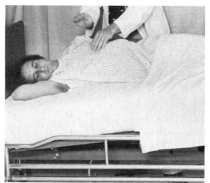

6 To drain the superior and inferior segments of the lingula, elevate the foot of the bed 15°. Position your patient so he's lying partly on his back and partly on his right side. Place a pillow under his left side for support. Then percuss the left side of his chest between the fourth and sixth ribs. To locate these, feel just above and below the nipple line.

CONTINUED ON PAGE 66

C.O.P.D. MANAGEMENT CONTINUED

PERFORMING CHEST PHYSIOTHERAPY CONTINUED

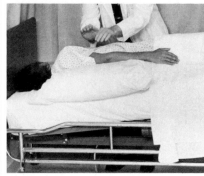

7 To drain the middle lobe of the right lung, raise the foot of the bed 15°. Then position your patient so he's lying partly on his back and partly on his left side, as shown here. Place a pillow under his back for support. Now, percuss the right side of his chest between the fourth and sixth ribs.

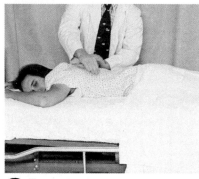

8 To drain the superior segments of both lower lobes, keep the bed flat. Position your patient on his abdomen. Then percuss both sides of his back over the lower ends of his scapulae.

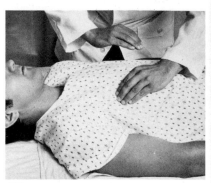

9 To drain the anterior basal segments of both lower lobes, elevate the foot of the bed 30°. Position your patient on his back, and percuss both sides of his chest. *Don't* percuss the center of his chest, over his stomach, since this could cause pain.

Important: An acutely ill patient may have trouble breathing in this position. If he does, adjust the bed angle to one he can tolerate. Then begin percussing.

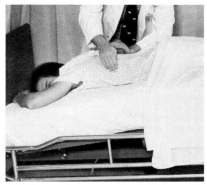

10 To drain the posterior basal segments of both lower lobes, raise the foot of the bed 30°. Position your patient on his abdomen. Percuss both sides of his back at the 10th-rib level and above, as shown here. To avoid causing pain, *don't* percuss over his kidneys, which are located below the 10th-rib level.

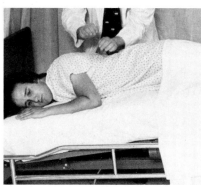

11 To drain the lateral basal segment of the left lower lobe, elevate the foot of the bed 30°. Position your patient so he's lying partly on his abdomen and partly on his right side, as shown here. Then percuss his left side at the 10th-rib level and above.

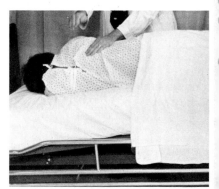

12 To drain the lateral basal segment of the right lower lobe, raise the foot of the bed 30°. Position your patient so he's lying partly on his abdomen and partly on his left side. Then percuss his right side, as shown here, at the 10th-rib level and above.

FOR THE PATIENT

EFFECTIVE BREATHING TECHNIQUES

To help prevent acute COPD episodes, learn to control your breathing by using either the abdominal or pursed-lip method. By practicing these methods regularly and using them during all your activities, you can keep your lungs free of stale air and gain confidence in managing your disorder.

Abdominal breathing

1 Lie comfortably on your back, with your knees bent, and relax your abdomen.

2 Next, press your hands (or place a book) lightly on your abdomen to create resistance.

3 Keeping your chest still, begin breathing abdominally. You're performing the technique correctly if your abdomen and hands (or book) rise as you breathe in and fall as you breathe out.

Pursed-lip breathing

1 Close your mouth and breathe in through your nose, taking a normal breath. (If you take too large a breath, you'll have to exhale much more air.)

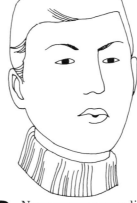

2 Now purse your lips as you would to whistle, and breathe out slowly through your mouth, without puffing your cheeks. Take at least twice the time you took to breathe in. Use your abdominal muscles to squeeze out every last bit of air you can.

3 During physical activity, always inhale before exerting yourself; exhale while performing the activity. For example, when walking up stairs, inhale between steps; exhale while climbing.

C.O.P.D. MANAGEMENT CONTINUED

INTERRUPTING AN ASTHMA ATTACK

To halt bronchospasm—the underlying cause of acute asthma—the doctor orders a bronchodilator, such as epinephrine or aminophylline. However, other supportive measures may also provide relief.

To help put asthma treatment in perspective, consider the case of 63-year-old Theresa Wolk, a retired bakery worker with a history of asthma. After experiencing tenderness in her left breast, Mrs. Wolk decided to see her gynecologist. During the examination, the doctor detected a small lump and scheduled a breast biopsy for the next day.

Frightened about the outcome of the biopsy, Mrs. Wolk had trouble sleeping that night.

Awakening the next morning, she felt short of breath, but she managed to get to the hospital without incident.

However, as you begin preparing her for the biopsy, she starts gasping for air. In a matter of seconds, she's wheezing, clutching at her neck to loosen her clothing, and using all her accessory muscles to breathe. Having just completed her patient history, you know she's asthmatic. With this in mind, together with your assessment findings, you decide she's having an acute asthma attack.

How to intervene. To give Mrs. Wolk the emergency care she needs, immediately place her in high Fowler's position and try to calm her down. Then call the doctor and prepare to take the following steps:

• Administer oxygen by nasal cannula or nasal prongs at 2 liters/minute until you can obtain arterial blood gas (ABG) measurements.

• Start an I.V. line of dextrose 5% in water to hydrate the patient. Most asthmatic patients are dehydrated from hyperventilation, profuse diaphoresis, and limited or no fluid intake. Administering I.V. fluid also helps liquefy the gel-like, tenacious sputum so your patient can clear the tracheobronchial tree. *Note:* Drugs are generally given parenterally to a patient having an acute asthma attack, since his airways are usually too clogged with mucus to benefit from aerosol administration.

• Administer subcutaneous serial injections of an adrenergic drug, such as epinephrine or terbutaline (Brethine).

• If bronchospasms persist, administer a parenteral methylxanthine drug, such as aminophylline.

• To treat possible bronchial inflammation, the doctor may also prescribe a corticosteroid, such as hydrocortisone or methylprednisolone. For complete details on COPD drugs, see the chart beginning on page 70.

• Have an arterial blood sample drawn to check ABG measurements. If your patient's receiving oxygen, note it on the laboratory slip.

• When ABG results arrive, adjust oxygen concentration appropriately to help the patient maintain PaO_2 in the 70 to 90 mm Hg range, if possible.

Pulmonary chair

This special chair, used by patients with asthma, emphysema, and pulmonary edema, improves total lung volume and vital capacity.

Drawing adapted with permission from Tampa Tracings, Tarpon Springs, Fla.

ARTERIAL BLOOD GASES: MAINTAINING A FINE BALANCE

Because a patient with chronic asthma compensates by hyperventilating during an acute episode, he usually maintains $PaCO_2$ at subnormal levels for years. However, don't assume every asthma patient always has a low $PaCO_2$ level. In some cases, a low $PaCO_2$ level may signal the start of further respiratory deterioration, possibly resulting in respiratory arrest.

Here's how an acute asthma attack goes from bad to worse: As the attack becomes more severe, the patient tires and his breathing slows. Consequently, his pH and $PaCO_2$ reach normal or near normal levels. However, as the attack continues, he becomes exhausted and begins to hypoventilate. His $PaCO_2$ level increases and his pH decreases, causing respiratory acidosis.

In many patients, respiratory acidosis precedes respiratory arrest. To prevent the sudden onset of respiratory acidosis, pay particular attention to serial ABG values. An abnormal progression like the one charted below indicates a respiratory imbalance leaning toward respiratory arrest. The patient will probably require endotracheal intubation, mechanical ventilation, and increased sedation, as ordered.

Special Note:

Respiratory acidosis inactivates epinephrine. Before administering this drug, give the patient sodium bicarbonate I.V. to help reverse acidosis and ensure epinephrine's effectiveness. (However, don't give sodium bicarbonate if the patient's ABG values reveal pH above 7.3 or bicarbonate above 20.) Administer sodium bicarbonate with oxygen, and carefully monitor the patient's serum potassium levels for hypokalemia.

Profile of a status asthmaticus attack

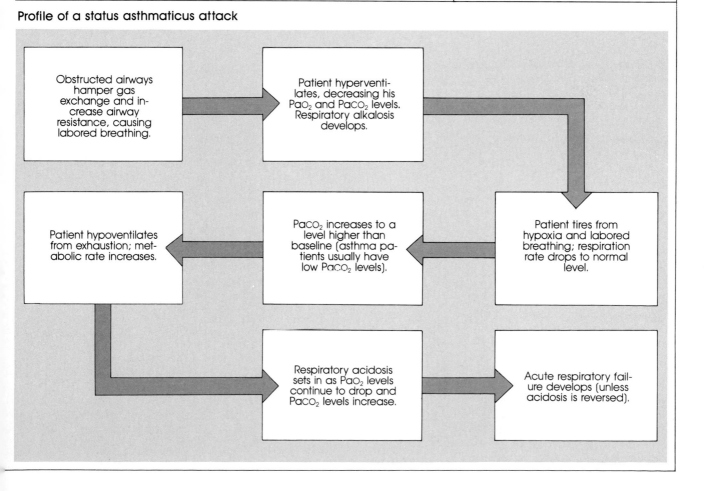

C.O.P.D. MANAGEMENT CONTINUED

STATUS ASTHMATICUS: A MEDICAL EMERGENCY

Although an acute asthma attack requires immediate care, it's usually reversible with proper treatment—or even reverses spontaneously. But if the asthma attack becomes prolonged and the patient fails to respond to standard therapy, you've got a medical emergency—status asthmaticus—on your hands.

In most cases, the severe bronchospasms that characterize status asthmaticus cause active and prolonged expirations. As bronchospasms worsen, pulmonary arterial pressure rises, causing the patient's neck veins to distend. Wheezing, a characteristic sign of asthma, may be absent if the airways become severely narrowed by the build-up of mucous plugs. Known as *silent chest*, this development portends respiratory arrest.

To avert this tragic outcome, move quickly to prevent complete bronchiolar obstruction. In most cases, the doctor will order standard treatment for reversing an asthma attack. If this fails, he'll probably instruct you to take the following measures:
• Administer metaproterenol or isoetharine hydrochloride 1% by nebulizer. (For details on nebulizer therapy, see page 64.)
• Give continuous drip I.V. aminophylline in a dosage based on the patient's age and weight, previous response to theophylline, recent drug history, and presence of cardiac disorders.
• Administer large doses of corticosteroids (for example, methylprednisolone may be given at 60 to 125 mg I.V. every 6 hours). These anti-inflammatory drugs not only promote bronchodilation and decrease bronchial edema, but they may also potentiate the actions of theophylline and adrenergic drugs.
• Closely monitor ABG values for signs of respiratory deterioration.
• Administer a broad spectrum antibiotic, such as ampicillin or tetracycline, if an infection precipitated the status asthmaticus episode.
• Because your patient could develop cardiac arrest momentarily, be prepared to intubate him and start mechanical ventilation if necessary.

As you provide the emergency care outlined here, keep the following important tips in mind:
• Don't confuse the tachycardia that commonly accompanies this condition with a dangerous dysrhythmia. Status asthmaticus tachycardia usually results from anxiety and sympathomimetic drug administration and requires no treatment.
• Because status asthmaticus is more severe than an ordinary asthma attack, the patient may be terrified. However, if he's been receiving a narcotic or sedative for pain or anxiety, withhold these drugs temporarily to avoid further depressing respirations.
• Don't risk alkalosis by hyperventilating the patient. To prevent this, have ABG values measured at regular intervals.

Special Note:

Identifying status asthmaticus in a patient with a known history of asthma is fairly easy. However, in a patient without such a history, don't mistake status asthmaticus for another chronic lung disease or pulmonary edema.

C.O.P.D. DRUGS

To achieve bronchodilation in a patient with acute respiratory failure, the doctor will probably order a drug combination that includes a xanthine derivative, a systemic corticosteroid, and an adrenergic. For details on these drugs, see the chart below.

XANTHINE DERIVATIVES
aminophylline, theophylline

Action:
Bronchodilation, smooth muscle spasm relief, increased ciliary action

Dosage:
Aminophylline
Loading dose: 6 mg/kg in 100 ml fluid over 20 to 30 minutes
Maintenance dose: 0.4 to 0.6 mg/kg/hour

Theophylline
100 to 200 mg P.O. every 6 hours; or extended-release form every 12 to 24 hours

Route:
Aminophylline: I.V.
Theophylline: P.O.

Adverse effects:
CNS: Irritability, insomnia, headache, restlessness, dizziness, convulsions (particularly with high dosages)
CV: Palpitations, sinus tachycardia, increased heart rate
GI: Loss of appetite, nausea, vomiting, gastric irritation
Other: Irritation from dehydration, muscle twitching

Nursing considerations:
Aminophylline and Theophylline:
• Contraindicated in patients with peptic ulcers, active gastritis, and hypersensitivity or idiosyncrasy to theophylline and other methylxanthines.

• Reduce dosage, as ordered, when administering to elderly patients or those with liver, kidney, or heart disease or a history of heavy smoking.
• Find out if the patient received theophylline therapy recently. The doctor may want to adjust the dosage.
• With plasma levels greater than 20 µg/ml, toxicity frequently occurs. Check the patient for signs and symptoms of toxicity, such as anorexia, nausea, vomiting, irritability, and headache.
• Don't administer with other drugs containing xanthine since severe toxicity may occur.

Aminophylline:
• Administer with an infusion pump, if available; or use a volume-control chamber.
• Monitor the patient's vital signs. Also check for cardiac dysrhythmias. If you detect a dysrhythmia, stop the infusion and call the doctor.
• Record the patient's intake and output.
• Check the I.V. site frequently to make sure the line's still in place.

Theophylline:
• To speed absorption, administer with a glass of water on an empty stomach; however, if the drug causes gastrointestinal irritation, administer with or immediately after meals.
• Don't substitute one brand of extended-release dosage form for another without the doctor's approval since the rate and extent of absorption varies among brands.
• Don't administer extended-release capsules as a loading dose.
• If your patient has difficulty swallowing the extended-release capsule, the contents may be mixed with or sprinkled on jam, jelly, or applesauce and taken without chewing.

CORTICOSTEROIDS
betamethasone, cortisone, dexamethasone, hydrocortisone, methylprednisolone, paramethasone, prednisolone, prednisone

Action:
Anti-inflammatory agent

Dosage:
Varies according to corticosteroid used

Route:
I.V. or P.O.

Adverse effects:
• Long-term use of corticosteroids in chronically ill patients can cause many side effects that can be minimized with alternate-day therapy. However, betamethasone and dexamethasone have a prolonged duration of action (more than 48 hours) and should not be administered this way.
CNS: Euphoria, insomnia, psychosis
CV: Congestive heart failure, hypertension, edema
EENT: Cataracts, glaucoma
GI: Peptic ulcer, GI irritation, increased appetite
Metabolic: Hypokalemia, hyperglycemia and carbohydrate intolerance, growth suppression in children
Skin: Delayed wound healing, acne, various skin eruptions
Other: Muscle weakness, pancreatitis, hirsutism, susceptibility to infections. Acute adrenal insufficiency may follow increased stress or abrupt withdrawal after long-term therapy.

Nursing considerations:
• Corticosteroids can impair white blood cell function in the lung, which may interfere with infection resistance.

• Because corticosteroids increase renal potassium excretion, monitor the patient's serum potassium levels closely. Potassium supplements may be necessary.
• Reduce dosage gradually after long-term therapy.
• Observe the patient for signs of infection.
• Weigh the patient daily, and report any sudden gain to the doctor.

ADRENERGIC DRUGS
albuterol, epinephrine, isoetharine, isoproterenol, metaproterenol, terbutaline

Action:
Bronchodilation

Dosage:
Varies according to adrenergic drug used

Route:
I.V., P.O., subcutaneous, nebulizer inhalant device, or IPPB machine

Adverse effects:
CNS: Nervousness, tremor, headache, drowsiness
CV: Increased heart rate, palpitations
GI: Nausea, vomiting, muscle cramps
Other: Sweating

Nursing considerations:
• Contraindicated in patients with known hypersensitivity to sympathomimetic drugs and in children under age 12.
• Use cautiously in patients with diabetes, hypertension, heart disease, hyperthyroidism, or a history of seizures.
• Teach the patient how to use aerosol and mouthpiece.
• Elderly patients usually require a lower albuterol dose.

RESTRICTIVE LUNG DISEASE

RESTRICTIVE LUNG DISEASE: A CLOSER LOOK

Restrictive lung disease isn't a single disorder but a group of diseases that restrict lung expansion and prevent adequate pulmonary ventilation. Restrictive lung disease can be interstitial or extrapulmonary. In this section, we'll explain the difference between the two types and tell you how to care for a patient with either.

Although not all restrictive lung diseases are life-threatening, most have that potential. Infection poses the greatest threat to respiratory function in restrictive lung disease patients, because their lung expansion's limited and they can't cough productively. Secretions clog the airways, producing a ventilation-perfusion mismatch that can end in respiratory failure.

Interstitial lung disease. In about 70% of patients with interstitial lung disease, the underlying cause remains unknown. These disorders gradually destroy elasticity in the affected lung, causing it to become stiff and noncompliant.

Fluid and various inflammatory and immune effector cells accumulate within extravascular lung tissues and spaces. When this happens, interstitial collagen breaks down, gathers in the interstitial spaces, and becomes fibrotic. Stiff, fibrotic scar tissue replaces normal elastic tissue, decreasing lung compliance. These fibrotic changes primarily affect the alveolar walls but may spread to the bronchioles—presumably from the variable tension exerted on bronchioles by uneven elasticity.

In advanced interstitial disease, constricted fibrotic tissue may cause alveolar dilation. Dilated regions alternate with constricted fibrotic areas, giving the lung a honeycomb appearance. Fibrosis may also narrow the pulmonary capillaries, impair blood flow to the affected areas, and thicken the interlobar septa and visceral pleurae. As cells, fluid, or fibrotic tissue accumulates in the interstitial spaces, they widen the alveolocapillary membrane. Beginning on the next page, we describe pleural effusion, atelectasis, and pneumonia—three interstitial diseases you should consider emergencies.

Extrapulmonary lung disease. In these disorders, lung structure remains normal but lung expansion's reduced. The cause can be a neurologic, neuromuscular, skeletal, or pleural abnormality. *Neurologic and neuromuscular disorders* (for example, myasthenia gravis and Guillain-Barré syndrome). These disorders destroy respiratory muscle tone or function, preventing the muscles from contracting sufficiently to expand the lungs and ventilate the alveoli. Atelectasis sets in, causing further lung stiffening. *Skeletal disorders* (for example, pickwickian syndrome and kyphoscoliosis). These may increase thoracic cage rigidity, reducing chest wall compliance and restricting lung expansion. *Pleural disorders* (for example, pleural effusion, pneumothorax, and hemothorax). These diseases can also restrict lung expansion. When the pleurae become inflamed, inspiration's so painful that the patient takes shallow breaths to avoid discomfort. Eventually, shallow breathing can lead to hypoventilated alveoli.

Differentiating restrictive from obstructive disease

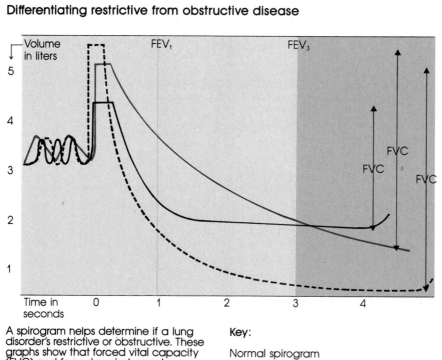

A spirogram helps determine if a lung disorder's restrictive or obstructive. These graphs show that forced vital capacity (FVC) and forced expiratory volume (FEV) decrease in restrictive disease. In obstructive disease, all parameters are reduced because the patient takes a longer time per unit to exhale.

Key:

Normal spirogram

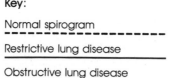

Restrictive lung disease

Obstructive lung disease

PLEURAL EFFUSION

PLEURAL EFFUSION: WHEN LUNG FLUID ACCUMULATES

The pleural cavity, a potential space between the parietal and visceral pleurae, holds only 20 ml of fluid at any given time. Yet several hundred milliliters of fluid pass through it daily. If fluid accumulates, pleural effusion develops.

Pleural effusion usually results from an abnormal change in the dynamics of pleural fluid transport, which causes the fluid production rate to exceed the removal rate. This change may reflect increased permeability of parietal pleural capillaries, increased hydrostatic pressure, altered colloid osmotic pressure, or reduced lymphatic drainage.

For example, increased capillary permeability in the parietal pleura commonly results from inflammation, either through pleural capillary damage or through histamines and other products of inflammation or cancer. Excess pleural fluid enters the pleural cavity, taxing the reabsorptive capacity of the visceral pleura and the lymphatic system.

A pleural effusion may be a hemothorax, a hydrothorax, a transudate, or an exudate.

Hemothorax. In this effusion type, blood enters the pleural cavity from rupture of the heart, great vessels, lungs, or chest wall vessels. Hemothorax usually follows blunt or penetrating chest trauma. For more information about this disorder, read the section beginning on page 120.

Hydrothorax. Treatment or diagnostic procedures cause this effusion type. For example, a displaced central venous catheter allows serum, intravenous hyperalimentation, or other intravenous fluid to enter the pleural cavity.

Transudative effusion. This fluid forms when pulmonary venous pressure rises or serum protein levels decrease. Most protein is filtered out as the fluid passes across the semipermeable parietal pleura.

Diseases that can cause transudative effusion include congestive heart failure, hepatic disease with ascites, hypoalbuminemia, or any disorder that overexpands intravascular volume.

Exudative effusion. An exudative effusion, in which poorly filtered, protein-rich fluid exudes into the pleural cavity, develops when capillary permeability increases or lymphatic drainage is blocked. Such effusions can result from inflammation, tuberculosis, subphrenic abscess, pancreatitis, cancer, pulmonary embolism, collagen vascular disease, myxedema, or chest trauma.

Types of exudative pleural effusions include empyema, chylothorax, pseudochylous effusion, and sterile exudates. Each type has a different composition, which can provide a clue to the underlying disorder.

Empyema, indicating pus, most often is related to pneumonitis, metastasis, or esophageal perforation or rupture.

Chylothorax, indicating chyle (digested triglycerides), results from trauma, thoracic duct disease, or lymphoma.

Pseudochylous effusion, signifying excessive amounts of cholesterol, is caused by cell degeneration.

Sterile exudates result from noninfectious inflammation, for example pancreatitis, cancer, pulmonary embolism, or collagen vascular disease.

RECOGNIZING SIGNS AND SYMPTOMS

A patient with pleural effusion may complain of various signs and symptoms. The most common complaint is chest pain so severe that he fears he's having a heart attack. Such pain may even give rise to other symptoms, depending on the effusion's extent and the patient's pulmonary status. Signs and symptoms to watch for are listed here:
• dyspnea; may indicate minimal lung collapse
• sharp stabbing chest pain aggravated by coughing or deep breathing (such as during exertion); relieved by short, shallow breaths and splinting; may radiate to neck, shoulders, or abdomen (since pain arises in intercostal nerves)
• shortness of breath (possibly from severe pain)
• dull or flat percussion, especially over the effusion
• absent or diminished voice sounds
• absent or diminished breath sounds over affected areas
• displaced heart sounds; may indicate mediastinal shift
• gallop heart rhythms; may indicate heart failure, frequently causing or accompanying effusion
• hypoxia secondary to underlying respiratory disorders or lung compression
• reduced lung volumes and areas of ventilation-perfusion mismatch.

Also check the patient's chart for any of the following factors that may predispose him to pleural effusion:
• preexisting fever, malaise, or purulent sputum
• a history of cardiac, hepatic, or renal disease
• recent drug therapy with hydralazine, methysergide, nitrofurantoin, or procainamide.

PLEURAL EFFUSION CONTINUED

ATELECTASIS

PLEURAL EFFUSION CARE: SETTING PRIORITIES

Suppose your patient's signs and symptoms suggest pleural effusion, and his chest X-rays reveal a density in his pleural space. What's the next step?

To confirm pleural effusion, the doctor will probably order a decubitus X-ray, then perform thoracentesis using the equipment pictured below before beginning antibiotic therapy. (See

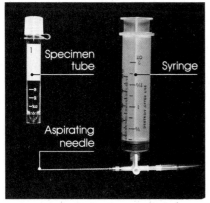

page 39 for information about your role in thoracentesis.) In the meantime, follow the nursing actions as outlined below, keeping in mind that treatment of pleural effusion's aimed at promoting ventilation and alleviating pain.

Promote adequate oxygenation.
• Raise the head of the patient's bed to a 45° angle (unless contraindicated).

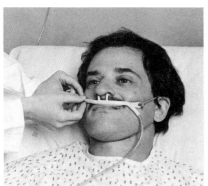

• Administer humidified oxygen, as ordered, if he has signs or symptoms of oxygen deficiency:

pallor, cyanosis, diaphoresis, confusion or change in level of consciousness, altered blood pressure, or increased heart or respiratory rate. (See pages 92 and 93 for details on oxygen therapy.)

Caution: Never administer oxygen to a COPD patient at a flow rate faster than 2 liters/minute.

Promote patient comfort.
• Advise him to lie on the affected *side,* and show him how to splint the painful area when coughing or breathing deeply.

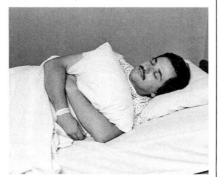

• Teach him to cough productively.
• Administer anti-inflammatory and analgesic drugs as ordered. Contact the doctor if pain persists. *Note:* Narcotics can diminish the cough reflex and slow respiration. If signs of respiratory depression develop, contact the doctor immediately.
• Raise the head of the patient's bed, or encourage him to sit up as much as possible. Both positions relax chest and abdominal muscles and make coughing less laborious.
• Relieve cough by administering antitussives as ordered.
• Discourage smoking.
• Use a vaporizer if necessary to maintain room humidity.
• Relieve his anxiety and provide emotional support by explaining the disorder and treatment. Encourage him to ask questions, and keep him and his family informed about his progress.

ATELECTASIS: WHEN ALVEOLI COLLAPSE

Atelectasis—the collapse of alveoli clusters or even an entire lung—commonly precedes a nosocomial respiratory infection. Yet atelectasis may appear as the end result of an infection.

By reducing the lung surface area available for effective gas exchange, atelectasis leads to intrapulmonary shunting and, ultimately, to hypoxia. To understand how this happens, first review the three major causes of atelectasis.

Ineffective ventilation. The most common cause of *postoperative atelectasis,* ineffective ventilation, stems from postoperative hypoventilation. You'll recall that after surgery, especially an abdominal procedure, a patient with incision pain may be afraid to breathe deeply. Instead, he takes shallow breaths, decreasing airflow and causing pooling of secretions in the alveoli.

Compressed alveoli from such disorders as abscess, pleural effusion, pneumothorax, or hemothorax can also reduce airflow and cause *compression atelectasis.* In severe viral or bacterial infection, atelectasis may develop from inflammation of the alveoli, capillaries, and interstitium.

Airway obstruction. An airway obstructed by a mucous plug or foreign body can cause *absorption atelectasis.* Trapped air distal to the obstruction diffuses into pulmonary circulation faster than it can be replaced by newly inspired air. Alveoli shrink and collapse. If lung tissue isn't pliable, tremendous negative pressure from extensive alveolar collapse draws fluid out of the pulmonary interstitium into the alveoli. Edematous alveoli then can cause atelectasis to spread to the entire lung.

Insufficient surfactant. Whether

The atelectatic alveolar unit

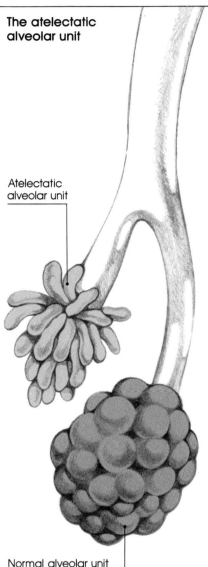

Atelectatic
alveolar unit

Normal alveolar unit

In a normal alveolar unit, air-filled alveoli exchange oxygen and carbon dioxide with capillary blood. In atelectasis, an airless, shrunken alveoli can't take part in gas exchange.

insufficient surfactant is a cause or an effect of atelectasis is unclear. Normally, surfactant coats the alveolar lining, reducing surface tension and preventing alveolar collapse during exhalation. Decreased production or inactivation of surfactant may contribute to alveolar collapse.

POSTOPERATIVE HYPOVENTILATION: AN OUNCE OF PREVENTION

A patient who's just out of surgery may find deep breathing painful or difficult. Unless you intervene, he could develop postoperative hypoventilation, a complication that can lead to atelectasis or pneumonitis. To encourage your patient to breathe normally, follow these guidelines:

Before surgery:
• Carefully evaluate the patient's history and clinical condition to detect factors that may predispose him to postoperative hypoventilation: lung disease, smoking, productive cough, shortness of breath, low exercise tolerance, heart disease or MI, or obesity. *Note:* If the patient greatly risks postoperative hypoventilation, the doctor may want to place him in the ICU after surgery.

After surgery:
• Check with the doctor before administering drugs or increasing dosages of drugs that can cause respiratory depression.
• Provide emotional support. If your patient fears incision pain so much that he hesitates to move, try to allay his fears by explaining the importance of turning periodically. Establish a turning schedule for the patient to follow.
• Teach him proper techniques for deep breathing, coughing, and splinting. If he needs incentive spirometry exercises, teach him how to use the equipment (unless a respiratory therapist is available).

INCENTIVE SPIROMETRY: FLOW VERSUS VOLUME

An incentive spirometer—a handheld, patient-operated device used to prevent such pulmonary disorders as atelectasis and pneumonia—can also help the patient who already has atelectasis. Properly used, the incentive spirometer reinflates collapsed alveoli, helps mobilize secretions, and measures the effort needed to sustain maximal inspiration.

Flow-incentive spirometer. This device measures how much airflow the patient generates during inspiration. This spirometer requires the patient to inhale through a vent for at least 3 seconds at a specific flow rate measured in cubic centimeters per second. If the patient generates an adequate flow rate, one or CONTINUED ON PAGE 76

Using an incentive spirometer

When used regularly, an incentive spirometer like the one shown below helps prevent atelectasis and other postoperative complications. The patient exhales normally, then inhales deeply through the mouthpiece until the balls rise to the chamber tops.

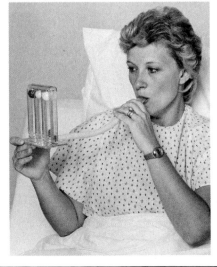

ATELECTASIS CONTINUED

INCENTIVE SPIROMETRY: FLOW VERSUS VOLUME
CONTINUED

more balls float upward inside a plastic chamber. For example, to elevate one ball, a patient must generate a 600-cc/second flow; two balls require a 900-cc/second flow; three balls, a 1,200-cc/second flow.

Volume-incentive spirometer.
This device calculates air volume from flow. As the patient inhales through the spirometer's mouthpiece, he draws air from a cylinder. If his inspiration's adequate, a piston rises to a preset level. This spirometer measures respiration more precisely than the flow-incentive spirometer; however, the patient shouldn't use it without assistance.

A deep breath held for a few seconds prevents pulmonary complications more effectively than multiple deep breaths that are immediately exhaled.

Nursing considerations. When deciding which spirometer's best for your patient, consider his age. Flow-incentive spirometers with ranges below 145 cc/second are best for pediatric and geriatric patients who commonly lack inspiratory force.

In most cases, spirometry exercises should be performed at least eight times daily to prevent atelectasis or hypoventilation. Although a respiratory therapist will probably explain the procedure to the patient and assist him with the exercises, make sure you're available to help.

YOUR ROLE IN I.P.P.B. THERAPY

To prevent or treat atelectasis, the doctor may order IPPB—intermittent positive-pressure breathing.

Although IPPB was once the keystone of pulmonary therapy, its routine use is now controversial. Its opponents argue that the treatments are costly and complicated and could easily be replaced with a hand-held nebulizer and deep-breathing exercises. However, IPPB therapy is still used in many institutions.

Usually administered for 15- to 20-minute periods several times a day, IPPB helps expand the airways, loosen secretions, and distend the tracheobronchial tree. By enhancing blood flow and distribution of inspired oxygen, it also improves the ventilation-perfusion balance.

Although a respiratory therapist usually sets up the equipment and supervises the patient during treatment, you'll prepare the patient and periodically evaluate his progress. Use the following guidelines to help your patient get the most out of IPPB therapy:

Before IPPB treatment:
• Have the patient sit in a chair with both feet on the floor. If he's

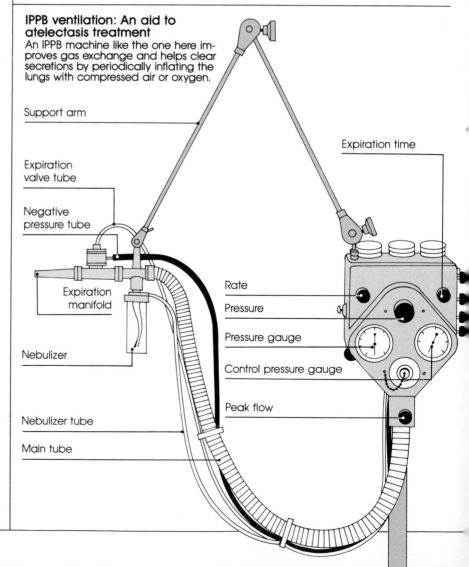

IPPB ventilation: An aid to atelectasis treatment
An IPPB machine like the one here improves gas exchange and helps clear secretions by periodically inflating the lungs with compressed air or oxygen.

Support arm

Expiration valve tube

Negative pressure tube

Expiration manifold

Nebulizer

Nebulizer tube

Main tube

Expiration time

Rate

Pressure

Pressure gauge

Control pressure gauge

Peak flow

PNEUMONIA

confined to bed rest, place him in a high-Fowler position, or seat him on the edge of the bed with both feet supported. (Sitting upright allows optimal lung expansion.)
• Measure the patient's blood pressure and heart rate, and listen to his breath sounds for later comparison.
• Instruct him to practice breathing slowly and deeply through his mouth.

During IPPB treatment:
• Ask the patient to seal his lips tightly around the mouthpiece and inhale slowly, allowing the machine to do the work. When he exhales, have him breathe out around the mouthpiece. Assure him that the technique will become easier with practice.
• Repeat the procedure until the nebulizer cup is empty.
• Record the patient's blood pressure and heart rate regularly. If you notice that his blood pressure's suddenly increased or that his heart rate's risen by 20 or more beats/minute, stop the treatment and notify the doctor immediately.

After IPPB treatment:
• Have the patient expectorate into tissues or a specimen cup, or suction him as necessary. He may also need to expectorate or to undergo suctioning frequently during treatment.
• Listen to his breath sounds and compare them with baseline sounds to evaluate the treatment's effectiveness.

Special Note:

Make sure the IPPB nebulizer contains medication, saline solution, or sterile water to prevent the patient's airways from drying and to mobilize his secretions.

EXPLORING THE CAUSES

While recuperating from an abdominal-perineal resection, your patient, Robert Truitt, develops a high fever (103° F., 39.4° C.), pleuritic chest pain, a productive cough, dyspnea, and shaking chills. During auscultation, you hear fine rales.

Suspect early bacterial pneumonia, because Mr. Truitt has the four cardinal signs of this condition.

To make a diagnosis, the doctor must first determine where the pneumonia's located—in the distal airways and alveoli (as in bronchopneumonia); in the alveolar septa and alveoli (as in interstitial pneumonia and alveolitis); in a lung lobe (as in lobular pneumonia); or in an entire lung (as in lobar pneumonia). Then, through sputum analysis, he can identify the causative organism.

Microbiologic causes. Pneumonia can be caused by a bacterium, virus, fungus, protozoon, mycobacterium, mycoplasma, or rickettsia. (Bacterial pneumonia is the fifth leading cause of death in debilitated patients.)

After a patient's inspired, aspirated, or directly contacted the pneumococcal bacterium, he quickly develops alveolar inflammation and edema. Pulmonary capillaries become engorged with blood and white cells, causing stasis. As tissues in the alveolar-capillary membrane break down, alveoli fill with blood and exudate, resulting in atelectasis.

In severe bacterial infection, the lungs take on the heavy, liverlike appearance seen in acute respiratory distress syndrome (ARDS). In severe cases, a lung abscess may form, causing pus to fill the lung parenchyma. If the abscess affects the bronchi, pus drains into the trachea and produces purulent sputum.

Streptococcus pneumoniae

(pneumococcus, or *Diplococcus pneumoniae*) causes about 80% of community-acquired bacterial pneumonias. Fortunately, the pneumococcal vaccine can destroy 23 of the most common strains. *Staphylococcus aureus*, the second most common pathogen, accounts for most cases of postinfluenza pneumonia. This pneumonia type's frequently complicated by lung abscess and has a high mortality when accompanied by viral pneumonia. *Klebsiella pneumoniae*, a relatively rare pathogen that appears in less than 4% of bacterial pneumonias, has a mortality of 20% to 50%. Often associated with alcoholism, it may be complicated by lung abscess. *Legionella pneumophila*, a gram-negative bacillus, can cause fatal shock or respiratory failure. This bacterium has also been found in some patients with community-acquired pneumonia. In these patients, the consequences are less serious.

Viral infection frequently causes diffuse pneumonia. The infection first attacks epithelial cells in the bronchioles, causing interstitial inflammation and desquamation. Infection soon spreads to the alveoli, which fill with blood and fluid. In an advanced infection, a hyaline membrane may form. A patient with severe viral pneumonia may have signs and symptoms resembling ARDS.

Aspiration pneumonia can be caused by aspiration of gastric juices or hydrocarbons from CPR, choking, or surgical anesthesia that interferes with the gag reflex. Aspirated particles usually enter the right lung because the right bronchus is aligned closer to the trachea than is the left. Acidic gastric juices can directly damage the airways and alveoli, causing mucosal damage, pulmo-

CONTINUED ON PAGE 78

PNEUMONIA CONTINUED

EXPLORING THE CAUSES
CONTINUED

nary edema, hemorrhage, and alveolar flooding. The more acidic a fluid is, the more damaging it is. Particles in aspirated gastric juices can also obstruct the airways and reduce airflow. This in turn leads to pooling of secretions and atelectasis, predisposing the patient to secondary bacterial pneumonia.

Aspirated hydrocarbons also cause inflammation and inactivate surfactant over a large alveolar area to cause alveolar collapse.

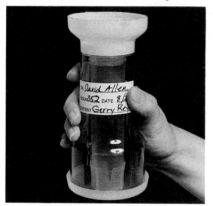

Sputum collection nursing tips. Does the doctor suspect your patient has pneumonia? To identify the pathogen, he'll order a sputum analysis. Keep the following points in mind while collecting the sputum specimen:
• If possible, collect the specimen first thing in the morning, after the patient brushes his teeth and rinses his mouth.
• Because the specimen must originate from the lungs, make sure the patient coughs deeply before expectorating. If you're using a suction catheter, make sure it extends to the bronchus.
• Collect at least 5 ml of sputum in a container like the one shown above to ensure accurate analysis.
• Send the specimen to the laboratory immediately.

FIGHTING THE INFECTION

After the doctor's identified the cause of your patient's pneumonia, he'll probably order one or a combination of several antimicrobial drugs. The chart below lists the drugs usually ordered for each pneumococcal bacterial infection. The doctor may also order an analgesic to relieve pleuritic pain and a bronchodilator to improve expectoration.

Also take these other supportive measures when caring for a pneumonia:
• Maintain adequate fluid intake.
• Encourage the patient to eat a high-calorie diet.
• Administer humidified oxygen to correct hypoxia (usually 4 to 6 liters/minute by nasal cannula or mask).
Note: If the patient's anemic, a blood transfusion may be ordered to restore oxygen-carrying capacity. If he has *severe* pneumonia, he'll probably be transferred to the intensive care unit for positive end-expiratory pressure (PEEP).

KLEBSIELLA
Drug therapy
Gentamicin, tobramycin, third-generation cephalosporins, or amikacin

LEGIONELLA
Drug therapy
Erythromycin

STAPHYLOCOCCUS
Drug therapy
Nafcillin, oxacillin, or first- or third-generation cephalosporins

STREPTOCOCCUS
Drug therapy
Penicillin G or first- or third-generation cephalosporins. Therapy can begin without waiting for specimen results.

CEPHALOSPORINS: THE THIRD GENERATION

Third-generation cephalosporins, which are being prescribed more frequently to treat pneumonia, also fight infections of the respiratory tract, skin, soft tissues, and genitourinary tract. Although the doctor may order one of these drugs as a penicillin substitute, administer them cautiously to patients with a known penicillin allergy. Such patients are five times more likely than other patients to develop an allergic reaction. Read the chart below for details:

CEFOTAXIME
Claforan*

Action
Antibacterial against gram-positive and a wide range of gram-negative organisms

Dosage
1 g I.V. or I.M. every 6 to 8 hours. In life-threatening infections, up to 12 g/day can be administered.

Adverse effects
Inflammation phlebitis and thrombophlebitis with I.V. injection; pain, induration, and tenderness after I.M. injection; maculopapular and erythematous rashes; urticaria; pruritus; fever; colitis; diarrhea; nausea; vomiting.

Special considerations
• Cefotaxime's contraindicated in patients with hypersensitivity to other cephalosporins. Use cautiously in patients with impaired renal function or penicillin allergy.
• Before therapy, obtain cultures for sensitivity tests.
• Administer cautiously in combination with probenecid to avoid cefotaxime toxicity.
• Monitor the patient carefully for superinfection.
• For I.V. use, reconstitute with at least 10 ml of sterile water for injection.

*Not available in Canada

MOXALACTAM
Moxam*

Action

Antibacterial activity against gram-positive and a wide range of gram-negative organisms.

Dosage

2 to 4 g I.V. or I.M. daily in divided doses every 8 hours for 5 to 10 days, or up to 14 days. In life-threatening infections or infections caused by less susceptible organisms, up to 12 g/day may be needed.

Adverse effects

Transient neutropenia; eosinophilia; hemolytic anemia; hypoprothrombinemia; bleeding; pain, induration, sterile abscesses, and tissue sloughing with I.M. injection; phlebitis and thrombophlebitis with I.V. injection; headache; malaise; paresthesia; dizziness; anorexia; nausea; vomiting; diarrhea; maculopapular and erythematous rashes; urticaria.

Special considerations

• Monitor bleeding time in patients receiving more than 4 g/day.
• If bleeding occurs and the prothrombin time is prolonged, promptly administer vitamin K.
• To prevent bleeding administer vitamin K (10 mg/week) prophylactically.
• Contraindicated in patients with hypersensitivity to other cephalosporins. Use cautiously in patients with impaired renal function or penicillin allergy.
• Before therapy, obtain cultures for sensitivity tests.
• Monitor the patient carefully for superinfection.
• For direct intermittent I.V. administration, add 10 ml of sterile water for injection, dextrose 5% injection, or 0.9% normal saline solution injection for each gram of moxalactam.
• Use cautiously in combination with probenecid to avoid moxalactam toxicity.

DRUG UPDATE

CEFOPERAZONE SODIUM: NEW ANTIPNEUMONIA WEAPON

A third-generation cephalosporin, cefoperazone (Cefobid*) was recently approved for treatment of pneumonia and other respiratory tract infections. For complete details on cefoperazone's actions, indications, and implications, read what follows.

Action

Antibacterial against gram-positive as well as a wide range of gram-negative organisms, including *pseudomonas*.

Dosage

1 to 2 g I.V. or I.M. every 12 hours. In severe infections or those caused by less sensitive organisms, total daily dosage may be increased to 16 g/day. I.M. doses should be injected deep into a large muscle mass, such as the gluteus or lateral aspect of the thigh.

Adverse effects

Transient neutropenia, eosinophilia, hemolytic anemia, hypoprothrombinemia, headache, malaise, paresthesia, dizziness, vomiting, diarrhea, pseudomembranous colitis, maculopapular and erythematous rashes, and urticaria. At injection site: pain, induration, sterile abscesses, temperature elevation, tissue slough. With I.V. injection: phlebitis, thrombophlebitis.

Special considerations

• Cefoperazone's contraindicated in patients with a hypersensitivity to other cephalosporins. Use cautiously in patients with impaired renal function or penicillin allergy.
• Before therapy, obtain cultures for sensitivity tests; however, therapy may begin pending test results.
• Prolonged use may result in an overgrowth of nonsusceptible organisms. Observe the patient carefully for superinfection.
• Use cautiously in combination with probenecid to avoid cefoperazone toxicity.
• Warn the patient to avoid alcohol for several days after discontinuing cefoperazone to avoid a disulfiram-like reaction.
• For I.V. use, reconstitute with dextrose 5% or 10% injection; dextrose 5% in Ringer's lactate; dextrose 5% in sodium chloride 0.2% or 0.9%; Ringer's lactate; sodium chloride 0.9%; Normosol-M and 5% Dextrose Injection; Normosol-R.
• Because of its rapid biliary excretion, cefoperazone's more likely than other cephalosporins to cause diarrhea.
• If bleeding occurs, administer vitamin K.
• Urine glucose determinations may be falsely positive with copper sulfate tests (Clinitest). Use Clinistix or Tes-Tape instead.

*Not available in Canada

RELATED CRISES

MYASTHENIA GRAVIS: HOW IT CAUSES RESPIRATORY FAILURE

Although myasthenia gravis is a neuromuscular disorder, it can also cause restrictive lung disease. (Guillain-Barré syndrome, another neuromuscular disease, can cause restrictive lung disease. In this syndrome, the myelin sheath covering the peripheral and cranial nerves is destroyed, causing sudden but reversible motor paralysis. For more information on this disorder, see NURSING NOW NEUROLOGIC EMERGENCIES.)

Myasthenia gravis produces sporadic but progressive weakness and fatigability of skeletal muscles. It takes an unpredictable course, with periods of remission sion alternating with exacerbations. Although the cause is unknown, failure of nerve impulse transmission at the neuromuscular junction results.

Myasthenia gravis can affect any muscle group. However, it usually first strikes muscles innervated by cranial nerves, then progresses to other areas. If it affects the respiratory muscles, it can be fatal.

Intervention. To help curb muscle weakness, you'll administer anticholinesterase drugs, such as neostigmine (Prostigmin) and pyridostigmine (Mestinon). As the disease worsens, however, these drugs become less effective, and the doctor may then order corticosteroids.

Crisis. Respiratory failure can occur during a *myasthenic* or *cholinergic* crisis. In myasthenic crisis, severe generalized muscle weakness develops suddenly, paralyzing the respiratory muscles. This emergency usually results from inadequate levels of the anticholinesterase drugs used to treat the disease. These drugs mimic the action of acetylcholine, which triggers skeletal muscle contraction.

Cholinergic crisis, which produces similar symptoms, usually results from overmedication.

Signs and symptoms. Some symptoms are common to both crisis types. These include generalized weakness with difficulty breathing, swallowing, chewing and speaking; increased salivation, lacrimation, bronchial secretions, and sweating; and apprehension and restlessness.

However, only myasthenic crisis produces the following symptoms:
• sudden, marked rise in blood pressure
• increased pulse rate
• absence of cough and swallow reflexes
• bladder and bowel incontinence
• severe cyanosis
• decreased urine output.

Cholinergic crisis produces these distinguishing symptoms:
• abdominal cramps and diarrhea
• muscle twitches
• nausea and vomiting
• blurred vision.

Distinguishing crisis types. An edrophonium (Tensilon) test can distinguish myasthenic from cholinergic crisis. If the patient regains muscle function within 1 minute after receiving edrophonium by I.V. infusion, he's in myasthenic crisis. (Improvement lasts no longer than 10 minutes, however.) A patient in cholinergic crisis will become even weaker after an edrophonium injection.

Managing a crisis. The doctor may order increased doses of cholinergic drugs for a patient in myasthenic crisis who responds positively to edrophonium infusion. Suctioning may also be needed to control secretions. If respiratory muscle paralysis is acute, an emergency airway or tracheotomy and mechanical ventilation may be necessary.

The doctor will withhold cholinergic drugs for a patient in cholinergic crisis. Keep a syringe containing 1 mg of atropine sulfate close at hand, since this dose may need to be injected I.V. to counteract severe reactions.

Preventing a crisis. To help the patient minimize exacerbations and complications, take the following nursing measures:
• Establish the patient's baseline respiratory and neurologic status.
• Monitor his tidal volume and vital capacity regularly.
• Stay alert for indications of an impending crisis.
• Administer drugs at the proper intervals.
• Teach the patient that strenuous exercise, stress, infection, and unnecessary exposure to cold or sunlight can worsen symptoms.
• Help him plan daily activities to coincide with energy peaks.
• Stress the need for frequent rest periods.
• Warn him that he should expect periodic remissions and exacerbations.

Neuromuscular junction: Weak link in myasthenia gravis

In myasthenia gravis, some nerve impulses can't cross the neuromuscular junction (indicated by arrow below).

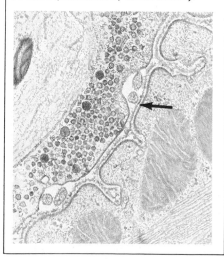

OXYGENATION DISORDERS

EMBOLISM BASICS

EMBOLISM MANAGEMENT

A.R.D.S.

NEAR DROWNING

TOXIC CHEMICAL
INHALATION

EMBOLISM BASICS

PULMONARY EMBOLISM: A REVIEW

Pulmonary embolism (PE) frequently complicates the recovery of hospitalized patients. Each year, half a million Americans develop it during a hospital stay. Yet PE usually can be anticipated or even prevented by good nursing care. In this section, we'll show you how to provide this care by explaining:
• how an embolism can grow from a simple blood clot in the pelvis or thigh to an obstruction that impedes blood flow to the lungs and imperils a patient's life
• how to assess PE's often obscure signs and symptoms
• how to identify the high-risk patient and which nursing steps you can take to help minimize this risk.

Embolus formation. PE begins when a solid mass lodges in a branch of the pulmonary artery, partially or completely obstructing the artery. The mass may be bone, air, fat, amniotic fluid, or a foreign object that's found its way into the vascular system (for example, needle or catheter parts).

In most cases, though, the invading substance is a blood clot, or thrombus, dislodged from a vein or the heart. Most emboli evolve from deep vein thrombi of the pelvis or thigh.

A thrombus sometimes dissolves on its own. But in response to direct trauma, abrupt muscle action, or changes in intravascular pressure, it may loosen or fragmentize. Once dislodged, the thrombus floats to the right side of the heart, then enters the lung through the pulmonary artery. Here, the mass (now termed an embolus) may dissolve or continue to fragmentize.

But emboli frequently grow rather than dissolve or fragmentize. The bigger the embolus, the more critical the patient's condition. Should it grow large enough to clog most or all of the pulmonary vasculature, it could be fatal.

A hazardous progression. Cut off from access to blood flow, air in the embolized lung zone (usually a wedge-shaped region) can't participate in gas exchange. Ventilation exceeds perfusion, creating physiologic dead space, which can produce arterial hypoxia. In massive PE, half or more of the vascular bed is lost, sharply increasing pulmonary vascular resistance.

Normally, only about 10 mm Hg of pressure's needed to pump blood through the pulmonary vasculature. But when vascular resistance is abnormally high, as it is in PE, pulmonary circulatory pressure increases to overcome resistance and adequately perfuse the lungs. To maintain such high pressure, the heart's right ventricle must pump harder. If the ventricle can't generate sufficient arterial pressure to maintain adequate cardiac output, ventricular failure occurs. Untreated, the patient's almost

sure to develop cardiac arrest. About 70% of patients with massive PE die within the first hour.

PE can provoke two other events: pulmonary hemorrhage and pulmonary infarction. In hemorrhage, red blood cells and plasma fill the affected lung zone, producing congestion that may cause hemoptysis.

If an embolism totally obstructs the arterial blood supply, pulmonary infarction, or lung tissue death, occurs. Approximately 10% of patients with PE develop this condition.

Other consequences. PE can cause atelectasis. Robbed of their normal blood supply, alveoli can't manufacture enough surfactant to keep from collapsing. Poor ventilation in embolized lung areas contributes to the problem.

Pulmonary edema may also develop. As right ventricular failure progresses, systemic venous pressure and hydrostatic pressure in peripheral veins mount, increasing permeability within pulmonary capillary membranes.

How the body fights back. Fortunately, most emboli aren't totally occlusive. And if total occlusion does occur, it usually lasts only a few hours. Through a mechanism called resolution, the body's fibrinolytic system tries to restore normal vascular flow by breaking down and dissolving the embolus. Resolution normally begins within hours of embolus formation, relieving PE's most acute effects.

Not every patient can complete the resolution process. But the patient who can't has other defenses. His body begins a process called organization to incorporate the damaged area into the affected vessel's lining. If successful, either process—resolution or organization—takes 7 to 10 days to resolve the embolus.

How an embolus develops
An embolus begins as a thrombus. As it grows, the thrombus may obstruct the blood vessels or fragmentize (as shown in the illustration below), producing emboli that may travel to the lungs.

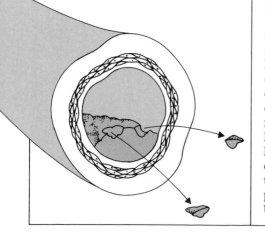

WHO'S AT RISK

What makes the hospitalized patient so at risk of developing PE? First of all, the reason he was hospitalized may be a contributing factor. Surgery, for example, promotes blood stasis, and anesthesia inevitably injures some lung vessels. Prolonged bed rest or pain can compound the risk by immobilizing the patient and encouraging stasis.

Other factors include venous injury, stasis, disease, increased blood coagulability, and the patient's age (if he's over 40).

Conditions that can cause venous injury:
• surgery, particularly on the legs, pelvis, abdomen, or thorax
• fractures or injury of the legs or pelvis
• I.V. drug abuse

Conditions that promote stasis:
• prolonged bed rest or immobilization
• obesity
• advanced age
• burns
• postpartum period

Diseases that put patient at higher risk:
• lung disease, especially chronic
• heart disease
• infection
• diabetes mellitus
• history of thromboembolism, thrombophlebitis, or vascular insufficiency
• polycythemia

Conditions that increase blood coagulability:
• cancer
• use of high-estrogen oral contraceptives

YOUR ROLE IN PREVENTING PULMONARY EMBOLISM

You play a pivotal role in preventing PE, a condition that can threaten nearly every hospitalized patient. To do so, include in your nursing care these preventive measures for promoting peripheral circulation:
• Encourage early, frequent ambulation (unless the patient's confined to bed for other reasons).
• If the patient's bedridden, turn him frequently and assist him with passive range-of-motion leg exercises.
• Elevate his legs 15 degrees. However, avoid using the bed's knee gatch, since popliteal pressure could help form a clot.
• Apply elastic antiembolism stockings or inflatable boots, as ordered, to augment venous pressure. If the doctor doesn't order these measures, remind him. When applying stockings, make sure they fit properly. If they're wrinkled, twisted, or too tight, they could cause thrombophlebitis. If they're too loose, they're ineffective.
• Don't let the patient sit for more than an hour. Provide a footstool, so he can extend his legs while sitting.
• For a high-risk patient, be prepared to administer prophylactic heparin, as ordered, to help prevent thrombus formation. If the doctor fails to order heparin, discuss your concerns with him.
• Avoid doing anything that may cause a clot to loosen and enter the bloodstream. For example, don't rub or massage the legs of a high-risk patient. Also, don't let him do isometric exercises or abruptly dangle his legs over the side of the bed, since either could cause a sudden change in blood flow to the legs.

Thwarting thrombosis and embolism: Another option

Continuous passive-motion devices, such as the Sutter CPM shown below, help to prevent venous thrombosis after certain surgical procedures. The machine's cyclic pumping action improves venous blood flow.

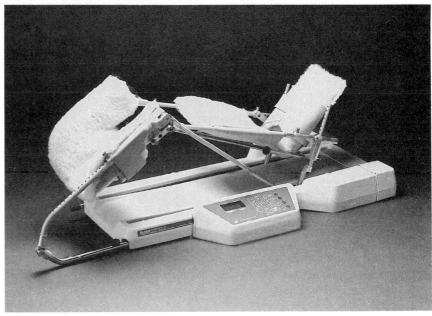

EMBOLISM BASICS CONTINUED

USING THE VENODYNE INTERMITTENT COMPRESSION SYSTEM

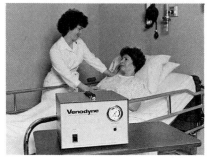

1 For a patient at risk of developing PE, the doctor may order Venodyne intermittent compression treatments, which help prevent thrombus formation by stimulating blood flow in the legs.

Explain the procedure to your patient, assuring her it's not painful. Tell her that she'll feel pressure on her legs as the vinyl pressure sleeves rhythmically inflate and deflate.

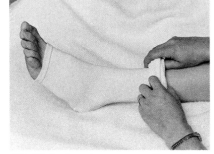

2 Help her into a comfortable position; then place a pillow under her knees, if possible. Pull the stockinets onto her legs, making sure they extend just above her knees. Smooth out any wrinkles.

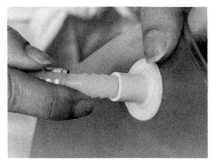

3 Push the other end of the tubing into the sleeves' input ports. (*Note:* If you're applying a pressure sleeve to one leg only, leave the unused sleeve attached to the system or clamp its hose to prevent air leakage.) Connect the end of the Y tubing to the VENODYNE OUTPUT CONTROL on the instrument's back panel.

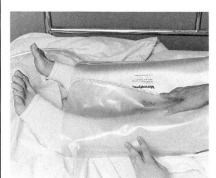

4 Press the vinyl sleeves flat to squeeze out any air. Make sure the sleeves are the correct size for your patient. Then slip them onto the patient's legs with the seam on top. Both ends of the stockinets should extend beyond the sleeves. Arrange the sleeves and tubing so that the sleeves will freely inflate.

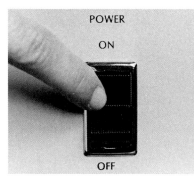

5 Turn on the power switch. Depress the PUSH TO TEST button on the back panel, and hold it until the gauge needle reaches the preset maximum ordered by the doctor (usually 40 to 45 mm Hg). If the gauge pressure rises slowly, check for air leaks.

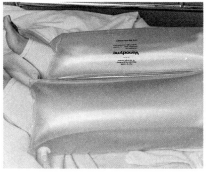

6 Release the PUSH TO TEST button. The pressure sleeves will automatically inflate and deflate in cycles, with inflation lasting about 12 seconds and deflation lasting about 48 seconds. At the end of the prescribed operating time, turn the power switch off and remove the sleeves and stockinets.

Caution: Intermittent compression is contraindicated for any patient with acute thrombophlebitis or deep vein thrombosis.

ASSESSMENT GUIDELINES

Assessing a patient with PE isn't easy. Signs and symptoms can be subtle or dramatic, mimicking various disorders such as anxiety and acute myocardial infarction.

How critically PE affects your patient depends largely on the degree of pulmonary arterial obstruction (determined by the size, number, and location of emboli). Cardiopulmonary status plays a part, too. A patient with a history of heart or lung disease may have relatively severe signs and symptoms.

Dyspnea. If your patient becomes acutely short of breath for no apparent reason, suspect PE. For many PE patients, dyspnea's the only complaint. Dyspnea's a sign that the body's attempting to compensate for impaired gas exchange. Breathing becomes labored as the patient tries to increase ventilation to lung areas unaffected by the embolism.

Three clinical portraits. The most common PE type is *simple PE,* in which less than half the pulmonary vascular bed is affected. Monitor the patient with simple PE for dyspnea, tachypnea, and tachycardia. Listen for rales or wheezing during auscultation. The patient may be apprehensive and may have an annoying cough, mild temperature elevation, pleural friction rub, and documented phlebitis. ABG values may show low PaO_2 and $PaCO_2$.

If your patient has progressive dyspnea, sharp pleuritic chest pain, or hemoptysis, he could have PE that's progressed to *pulmonary infarction.* You may hear pleural friction rub on auscultation.

Massive PE—obstruction of more than half the pulmonary vascular bed—produces worsening dyspnea, anxiety, hypoxia, severe hypotension, cardiac dysrhythmias, or cyanosis. Cardiac arrest may also occur.

Pulmonary embolism: Signs and symptoms

Use this illustration as a guide to assessing your patient who's at risk of developing pulmonary embolism.

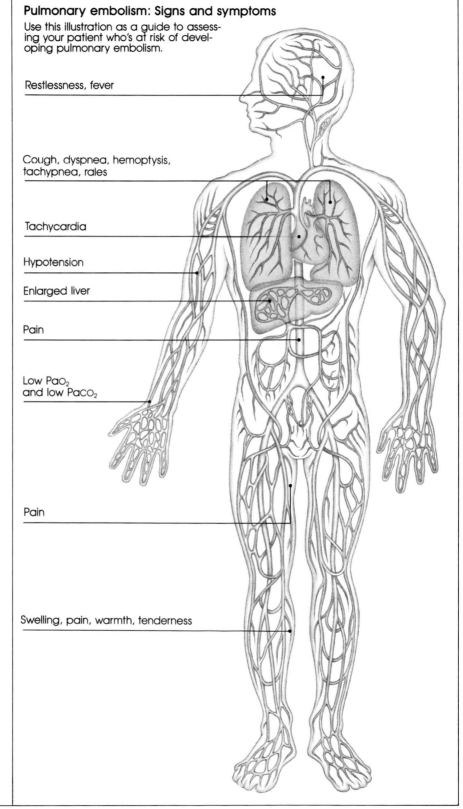

Restlessness, fever

Cough, dyspnea, hemoptysis, tachypnea, rales

Tachycardia

Hypotension

Enlarged liver

Pain

Low PaO_2 and low $PaCO_2$

Pain

Swelling, pain, warmth, tenderness

EMBOLISM BASICS CONTINUED

DRUG UPDATE

NEW DRUG APPROACH TO P.E. PREVENTION

An experimental approach to preventing PE combines low-dose heparin with an alpha blocker, dihydroergotamine mesylate (D.H.E. 45).

Researchers found that when given postoperatively in the proper dosages, this drug combination significantly reduced the venous thrombosis rate in high-risk patients.

Like other alpha blockers, dihydroergotamine constricts the veins, counteracting venous stasis and promoting venous return from the legs.

Just before surgery and for 5 to 7 days afterward, patients in five randomized groups received subcutaneous injections of one of the following: placebo, heparin, dihydroergotamine, or heparin with dihydroergotamine in one of three different dosage combinations.

In the group receiving 0.5 mg of dihydroergotamine plus 5,000 units of heparin, the venous thrombosis rate was 9.4%. In the group with the second lowest incidence (16.8%), each received the same dihydroergotamine dosage but half as much heparin as the first group. Almost 20% of patients receiving dihydroergotamine alone developed thrombosis.

DIHYDROERGOTAMINE MESYLATE (D.H.E. 45) WITH HEPARIN SODIUM (Hepalean**, Liquaemin Sodium*)**

Mechanism of action
Acts as an alpha blocker to prevent sympathetic stimulation; constricts veins and venules with minimal resistance of arteries and arterioles.

Dosage
0.5 mg of dihydroergotamine plus 5,000 units of heparin every 12 hours

Possible adverse effects
Hemorrhage, wound hematoma, decreased hemoglobin, irritation at injection site

Contraindications
Prolonged hypotension, overt infection, severe sepsis, shock

Special considerations
• Monitor hemoglobin levels and prothrombin times.
• Check injection site for irritation and hematoma.

*Not available in Canada   **Not available in the United States

---

AIR EMBOLISM: AN AVOIDABLE CRISIS

Is your patient receiving fluid or medication through a central venous catheter? Improper catheter insertion and removal—or even routine catheter care that's improperly performed—could cause an air embolism as life-threatening as any other type. Air embolism can also occur after open heart surgery or surgery of the head, neck, or peritoneal cavity.

Like a blood clot, an air bubble in a vein floats through the vena cava to the heart's right ventricle. From here it's pumped to the pulmonary vasculature, where it fragmentizes into many tiny bubbles that clog the pulmonary artery. Unless treated, the patient risks the same dangers as he would with thromboembolism: reduced cardiac output, ventricular failure, and cardiac arrest.

How much air in a vein is too much? Using animal studies, one researcher estimated that signs and symptoms of air embolism can occur when 20 cc of air per second enter a vein; 70 to 150 cc of air per second may be fatal.

Central venous line care. Before the doctor inserts the catheter, position the patient with his head lower than the level of the heart (Trendelenburg's position). Because intrathoracic pressure's greater in this position, air is less likely to be sucked into the vein when the patient inspires. (If your patient's hypovolemic, make sure his blood volume's increased before catheter insertion to avoid hypovolemia from intensifying the vein's sucking force.)

Have the patient perform Valsalva's maneuver during insertion. To do this, instruct him to hold his breath and then to bear down and tighten his throat muscles without exhaling.

Once the catheter's in place,

prevent it from contacting atmospheric air. To do this, make sure the connection between the tubing and catheter hub is tight—but not so tight that you might have to loosen it with an instrument that could crack the hub.

Secure the catheter to the patient to prevent the tubing from becoming dislodged as he shifts positions. Use a dressing small enough to permit you to check the connection easily. (Dislodgement's a particular risk with a jugular insertion site, so before allowing your patient to sit or stand, always check the catheter connections.)

When changing the tubing, place the patient in Trendelenburg's position and have him perform Valsalva's maneuver for the few seconds that the catheter's open (especially if he's dyspneic or critically ill).

Cover the insertion site with a petrolatum gauze occlusive dressing before catheter removal to prevent air from entering the catheter tract.

Intervention. If you suspect air embolism, immediately turn the patient onto his left side in the Trendelenburg position. This helps air bubbles float toward the heart's right atrium and away from the pulmonary artery, permitting blood to enter the lungs.

Usually, air bubbles disperse slowly through the pulmonary system. If not, the doctor may insert a catheter into the right atrium and try to remove the air.

DIAGNOSING PULMONARY EMBOLISM

Because PE can be so hard to diagnose, the doctor's evaluation process may become increasingly complex before he arrives at a conclusion. He may order most or all of the following tests, depending on the patient's signs and symptoms and each test's results:

Blood tests. These are used mainly to rule out other conditions. In a complete blood count for a patient with PE, you may find elevated white blood cells and sedimentation rate. Arterial blood gas (ABG) measurements may reveal arterial hypoxemia, indicated by a PaO_2 level of less than 75 mm Hg. The $PaCO_2$ value may rise in early PE, causing respiratory acidosis, then drop during later stages. *Note:* If your patient has preexisting cardiopulmonary disease, ABG values aren't reliable.

However, these results are common to some other conditions. A more valuable PE indicator is the *absence* of arterial hypoxemia. Only 6% of patients with PE have a PaO_2 level above 90 mm Hg.

EKG. PE doesn't cause specific EKG changes. But an EKG *can* determine if heart disease is the cause of your patient's chest pain. It may also show the following changes that suggest PE: tachycardia, disturbed rhythm, enlarged P waves, depressed ST segment, and inverted T waves. If your patient has massive PE, his EKG may show right axis deviation, a sign of right ventricular failure.

Chest X-ray. Even if your patient has a sizable embolus, his chest X-ray may be normal. In some cases, PE shows up as a high diaphragm on the embolized side, pleural fluid, enlarged pulmonary arteries, or abrupt cutoff of a pulmonary artery shadow. Obvious differences in major blood vessel diameters may reflect shunting of blood around alveolar dead space to areas supplied by dilated vessels. Tiny pulmonary infiltrates indicating atelectasis may be visible in some alveoli, particularly at the lung bases.

If infarction has occurred, a humped shadow (Hampton's hump) will appear on the infarcted areas.

Lung scintigraphy. The ventilation scan and lung perfusion scan are most useful when the results are compared. In both tests, radioactive material is absorbed into the body and its distribution pattern scanned to view lung function. When compared, results of the two scans may either rule out PE or suggest that it's likely.

Pulmonary angiography. This invasive study, using right-heart catheterization, is the most specific and conclusive diagnostic test for PE. Because this study is expensive and somewhat risky, it's done only when the doctor requires a definitive diagnosis, for example, when lung scintigraphy can't provide enough information about a critically ill patient. In this test two findings indicate certain PE: a filling defect in a pulmonary vessel and the abrupt ending of a vessel.

Special Note:

If the doctor suspects your patient has a PE, he may order 3,000 to 5,000 units heparin I.V. bolus every 4 hours to protect the patient during diagnostic studies. If the diagnosis is confirmed, heparin may either be continued or replaced with thrombolytic therapy. If PE's ruled out, heparin's discontinued immediately.

EMBOLISM BASICS CONTINUED

LUNG SCINTIGRAPHY

If your patient has signs and symptoms of PE, the doctor may order lung scintigraphy to help confirm the diagnosis. Consisting of complementary tests known as the lung perfusion scan and ventilation scan, scintigraphy yields valuable information about pulmonary blood flow and gas exchange. Both scans aren't performed in every case, but the tests are most useful when their results are compared.

Lung perfusion scan. Also called the lung scan or lung scintiscan, this test shows pulmonary blood flow. To produce this image, a radioactive agent is injected into a peripheral vein. A scintiscanner detects the pattern of radioactive uptake within the lung, then transfers it to an oscilloscope for display. From this image, the doctor can trace perfusion patterns.

A cold spot—an area of low radioactive uptake—indicates absent or decreased blood flow that could mean PE. If no cold spots appear, the doctor can rule out PE.

However, cold spots are no guarantee that the patient has PE. Pneumonia, atelectasis, and pneumothorax can also cause perfusion defects.

Ventilation scan. If cold spots appear on the perfusion scan, the doctor will probably order a ventilation scan, which delineates lung regions ventilated during respiration. For this test, the patient inhales air mixed with radioactive gas through a tight-fitting mask. A nuclear scanner records gas distribution during three phases. In the initial *wash-in phase*, gas is distributed through the airways. During the *equilibrium phase*, radioactivity reaches a steady level as the patient breathes room air from a bag. During the final *wash-out phase*, gas exits the lungs.

Normally, results show equal gas distribution in both lungs during wash-in and wash-out. Unequal distribution indicates poor ventilation or airway obstruction in areas with low radioactive uptake.

Comparing results. If an area with normal ventilation corresponds to a perfusion defect (cold spot), the doctor can probably assume the patient has PE.

If results show matched defects—areas where both ventilation and perfusion are poor—the patient probably has a parenchymal disease such as pneumonia, emphysema, or tuberculosis. (However, the doctor can't always rule out PE in this case, since an embolism can occur in lung areas where an underlying disease has compromised ventilation.)

Normal and abnormal lung perfusion scans

A normal lung with no perfusion defects appears in the lateral lung scan shown below. The lung outline is smooth, and the lung is uniformly dense, indicating normal radioactive uptake.

The lateral lung scan below shows uneven density resulting from a pulmonary embolus. Note the perfusion defects, or cold spots, caused by poor perfusion.

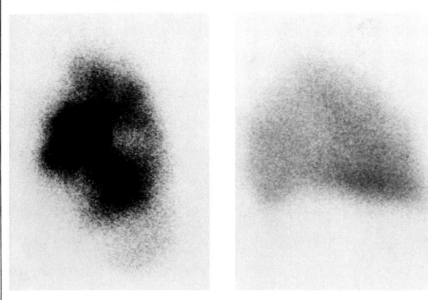

ULTRASOUND: FUTURE DIAGNOSTIC TOOL?

Researchers have found that an ultrasound device similar to an echocardiograph can effectively diagnose PE. The device measures parameters of pulmonary reflection and absorption.

To diagnose PE using ultrasound, researchers calculated three indexes: pulmonary reflection coefficient, tissue attenuation coefficient, and range-gated blood Doppler signals.

Combining these readings, the investigators detected 23 cases of PE among 25 patients whose embolism had already been confirmed by lung scintigraphy or pulmonary angiography.

Researchers believe this technique is more sensitive than lung scintigraphy. And unlike scintigraphy, it's apparently unaffected by COPD or other disorders.

DIAGNOSING P.E. THROUGH VENOUS THROMBOSIS SCREENING

Is your patient with suspected PE critically ill, pregnant, or hypersensitive to iodine, seafood, or radiographic dyes? If so, pulmonary angiography and lung perfusion scans may be too risky for diagnostic use. Instead, the doctor may try a different approach—venous thrombosis screening. The logic of this strategy is simple: 95% of patients with PE have deep vein thrombosis (DVT).

Three noninvasive techniques screen for DVT: impedance plethysmography, Doppler ultrasonography, and I^{125} fibrinogen scan. (Contrast venography, the radiographic examination of a vein, can also give definitive proof of DVT. But because it's invasive and somewhat hazardous, venography is usually contraindicated for patients who shouldn't undergo pulmonary angiography.)

Impedance plethysmography. This test measures venous flow in the legs. Electrodes from a plethysmograph are applied to the patient's leg to record impedance—changes in electrical resistance caused by blood volume variations. A pressure cuff wrapped around the patient's thigh is inflated to occlude venous circulation. If DVT is present, blood volume in leg veins below the cuff increases less than normally when the cuff is deflated, since these veins are already at capacity.

While impedance plethysmography is especially sensitive for DVT in the popliteal and iliofemoral veins, it's less accurate for calf-vein clots or partially occlusive thrombi.

Doppler ultrasonography. This method uses high-frequency sound-wave recordings to evaluate blood flow in the arms, legs, and neck. A hand-held probe called a transducer directs sound waves to the artery or vein being tested. After striking moving red blood cells, waves are reflected back to the transducer at frequencies corresponding with blood flow velocity through the vessel. (High-velocity blood flow produces high-frequency waves; low-velocity blood flow produces low-frequency waves.) The transducer amplifies and records the waves, enabling the doctor to listen directly to blood flow and view it graphically.

As measurements are taken, the patient changes position and performs breathing exercises to vary blood flow. Changes in sound-wave frequency during respiration help detect venous obstructions, since blood flow normally rises and falls with respiration. Blood pressure's checked at various sites to help detect the presence, location, and extent of arterial occlusive disease.

Doppler ultrasonography is about 95% accurate in detecting arteriovenous disease that obstructs at least 50% of blood flow. It may not detect smaller thrombi, however.

Radiofibrinogen scan. In this procedure, the patient's injected with radionuclide-labeled fibrinogen, a substance that collects at sites of active thrombus formation. A scintillation counter then records radioactivity at several calf and thigh sites at various time intervals.

If radioactivity increases more than 20% between adjacent sites on the same leg, compared with results of a previous scan, the patient probably has DVT. An abnormality persisting for longer than 24 hours confirms DVT.

The radiofibrinogen scan is most effective when preoperative and postoperative results are compared. It usually doesn't detect groin and pelvic thrombi because of high background radiation from large veins and arteries. Another drawback is that the test takes 24 hours to complete.

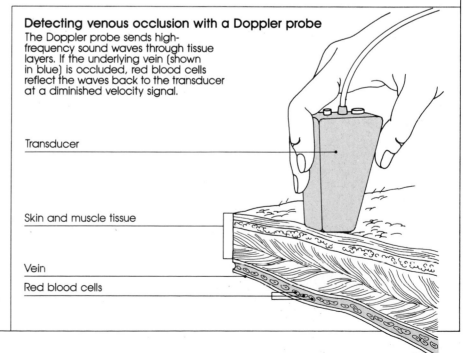

Detecting venous occlusion with a Doppler probe

The Doppler probe sends high-frequency sound waves through tissue layers. If the underlying vein (shown in blue) is occluded, red blood cells reflect the waves back to the transducer at a diminished velocity signal.

Transducer

Skin and muscle tissue

Vein

Red blood cells

EMBOLISM MANAGEMENT

TAKING IMMEDIATE STEPS

Does your patient have signs or symptoms of pulmonary embolism—for example, shortness of breath; increased heart rate; or rapid, shallow breathing? Don't delay intervention until the doctor can confirm the diagnosis.
Take the following steps immediately:
• Call for the doctor; then request that a respiratory therapist and another nurse be available for backup support.
• Make sure the patient's airway is clear.
• If he's having difficulty breathing, administer oxygen at a high-flow rate, if permitted by hospital policy.
• Establish an I.V. line. If a line's already in place, check its patency.
• Provide emotional support.
• Don't leave the patient's side until help arrives.
What to document. When documenting your patient's signs and symptoms or describing them to the doctor, you'll need to include the following information:
• time of onset
• rate, depth, and breathing effort
• use of any accessory muscles for breathing
• color of nail beds and mucous membranes. (Keep in mind, however, that cyanosis occurs only in late stages of PE.)
• breath sounds
• any change in cardiac status (for example, alterations in blood pressure, heart rate, or mental status; or neck vein distention)
• current oxygen therapy, if any.

ANTICOAGULANT THERAPY: DO'S AND DON'TS

Your patient with a pulmonary embolism is probably receiving heparin to reduce the risk of secondary thrombi (heparin can't dissolve an existing clot). Heparin therapy usually continues for 7 to 10 days. The doctor will probably order an oral anticoagulant such as warfarin a few days before heparin's discontinued. Warfarin takes 1 to 3 days to achieve therapeutic effect, although it alters prothrombin time (PT) the 1st day of therapy.

Review the following guidelines to help administer heparin and warfarin safely and effectively.

HEPARIN SODIUM
Hepalean**, Liquaemin Sodium*

Dosage and route
For continuous I.V. therapy: 5,000 to 10,000 units I.V. bolus; then 1,000 units hourly by I.V. infusion. (Some doctors may order a much higher loading dose.)

For intermittent therapy: 5,000 to 7,000 units I.V. push; then adjust the dose according to partial thromboplastin time (PTT) results.

Adverse effects
Excessive bleeding and hemorrhage; thrombocytopenia; local irritation or mild pain; hypersensitivity reactions (for example, chills, fever, pruritus, and rhinitis)

Nursing considerations
• Monitor PTT regularly. Anticoagulation is present when PTT values are 1½ to 2 times control values.
• Inspect the patient for bleeding gums, bruises, petechiae, nosebleeds, melena, hematuria, and hematemesis.
• When giving intermittent I.V. therapy, always obtain blood ½ hour before the next scheduled dose to avoid falsely elevated PTT.
• For continuous I.V. therapy, PTT should be taken any time after 4 to 6 hours of therapy. Never obtain blood for PTT from the I.V. tubing or from the infusion vein. Falsely elevated PTT will result.
• Avoid all I.M. injections.
• Never piggyback other drugs into an infusion line while heparin infusion is running. Some drugs inactivate heparin. Also, don't mix any drug with heparin in a syringe when administering bolus therapy.

WARFARIN SODIUM
Coufarin*, Coumadin, Panwarfin*

Dosage and route
10 to 15 mg P.O. for 3 days; then adjust the dose based on daily PT times (usual daily maintenance dose: 2 to 10 mg P.O.).

Adverse effects
Excessive bleeding and hemorrhage, increased menstrual flow, dermatitis, rash, fever, leukopenia, diarrhea, vomiting, nausea, fever

Nursing considerations
• Monitor PT regularly. Most doctors try to maintain PT at 1½ to 2 times normal. Bleeding may occur if PT exceeds 2½ times control values.
• Observe elderly patients and patients with renal or hepatic failure for exaggerated warfarin effect.
• Inspect the patient for bleeding gums, bruises, petechiae, nosebleeds, melena, hematuria, and hematemesis.
• The following drugs may increase the risk of bleeding when administered concurrently with warfarin: alcohol, acetaminophen (in high doses), androgens, chloral hydrate, cimetidine, clofibrate, disulfiram, metronidazole, oxyphenbutazone, phenylbutazone, quinidine, salicylates, and sulfonamides.
• The following drugs may reduce warfarin's therapeutic effect: barbiturates, carbamazepine, cholestyramine, colestipol, glutethimide, and rifampin.

*Not available in Canada   **Not available in the United States

PREPARING YOUR PATIENT FOR WARFARIN THERAPY

Does your patient require long-term warfarin therapy to prevent an embolism from recurring? Before he's discharged, take the following steps to ensure that his drug treatment remains effective and safe:

• Warn him to notify the doctor before taking any other medication, including aspirin and other over-the-counter products.

• Schedule him for regular outpatient laboratory tests, and stress the importance of keeping his appointments.

• Tell him to watch for and immediately report any bruising, unexplained bleeding, and signs of occult bleeding (for example, black or tarry stools, bloody urine, or coffee-ground vomitus).

• Encourage him to eat a consistent amount of leafy green vegetables every day. Otherwise, vitamin K levels could fluctuate, altering warfarin's anticoagulant effect.

• Tell him to take his medication at the same time every day and at the recommended dosage.

• Discourage unlimited intake of alcoholic beverages.

• Advise him to use an electric razor when shaving to avoid skin cuts, and to brush his teeth with a soft toothbrush.

• Give him a card identifying him as a potential bleeder, and advise him to carry it at all times.

FIBRINOLYTIC DRUGS: FAST-ACTING CLOT DISSOLVERS

If your patient has acute, massive PE, he'll need more than an anticoagulant, which merely prevents new clots from forming. In addition to other measures, his treatment will probably include streptokinase or urokinase—fibrinolytic drugs that can rapidly dissolve an embolus and reverse the accompanying severe complications.

Streptokinase and urokinase, natural proteins, hasten the body's clot-resolving mechanism by converting plasminogen to plasmin, which dissolves a clot's fibrin threads. These drugs begin to act immediately, sometimes resolving an embolus within 24 hours.

However, fibrinolytic drugs work indiscriminately and may dissolve even tiny blood clots. Because of the risk of hemorrhage, these drugs are contraindicated for patients with any of the following conditions: active or recent internal bleeding; surgery or other invasive procedures within the last 10 days; cerebrovascular accident within the last 2 months; pregnancy or recent obstetric delivery; severe hypertension; uncontrolled hypocoagulation; bacterial endocarditis or rheumatic valvular disease; acute or chronic renal or hepatic insufficiency.

STREPTOKINASE
Kabikinase*, Streptase

UROKINASE
Abbokinase*, Breokinase*

Dosage and route
Streptokinase
250,000 IU by I.V. infusion administered over 30 minutes; then 100,000 IU hourly by I.V. infusion for 24 to 72 hours
Urokinase
4,400 IU/kg by I.V. infusion administered over 10 minutes; then 4,400 IU/kg hourly by I.V. infusion for 24 to 72 hours

Adverse effects
Severe bleeding, decreased hematocrit, thrombophlebitis, anaphylaxis (streptokinase only)

Nursing considerations
• Use a volumetric infusion pump to administer the drug.

• Obtain baseline PT and PTT to determine the rate of I.V. infusion.

• Discontinue heparin and wait for effects to diminish before starting streptokinase.

• Keep aminocaproic acid (Amicar), packed red cells, and whole blood available for possible bleeding.

• Test all emesis, nasogastric aspirates, stool, and urine for blood. Notify the doctor if bleeding occurs.

• Inspect the dressing on the infusion site every hour for signs of bleeding. Apply direct pressure if bleeding occurs. Every hour check, compare, and document the pulses, color, and sensitivities of both arms.

• Monitor vital signs frequently.

• Withhold I.M. injections and keep venipunctures to a minimum for 24 hours after the infusion's complete.

• When the I.V. catheter's removed, apply direct pressure to the infusion site for at least 30 minutes.

Note: A patient allergic to streptokinase will suddenly develop dyspnea, bronchospasm, convulsions, cyanosis, or syncope. Stop the drug, call his doctor, and prepare to administer emergency drugs, as ordered.

*Not available in Canada

EMBOLISM MANAGEMENT CONTINUED

COMPARING OXYGEN DELIVERY SYSTEMS

Your patient with pulmonary embolism may need oxygen therapy to relieve and control dyspnea and hypoxia and to minimize the risk of cardiac complications. The doctor will choose either a low-or high-flow oxygen delivery system, depending on your patient's history and clinical condition. Each type can deliver both small and large concentrations of oxygen.

Low-flow systems (nasal cannula, simple face mask, partial rebreathing mask, nonrebreathing mask). These devices let the patient inhale room air, which mixes freely with oxygen. The concentration of oxygen delivered adapts to the patient's ventilatory pattern.

Although economical and comfortable, low-flow systems don't give a fixed oxygen concentration. They're the best choice for the COPD patient, who may need a hypoxic stimulus to breathe.

High-flow systems (devices using a venturi mask). Unresponsive to the patient's breathing pattern, these systems deliver exact oxygen concentrations. The venturi mask controls how much room air is entrained. High-flow systems are sometimes chosen for a patient with adult respiratory distress syndrome (ARDS).

To compare various oxygen delivery methods, study the chart on these pages.

Note: If your patient can't maintain an acceptable PaO_2 level or if he tires from persistent tachypnea while receiving oxygen, he may need mechanical ventilation, which controls oxygen concentration more effectively. On page 97, we describe the positive end-expiratory pressure (PEEP) and continuous positive airway pressure (CPAP) ventilation systems.

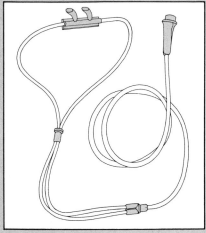

NASAL CANNULA
(low-flow system)

Benefits
• Safe and simple
• Comfortable; easily tolerated
• Effective for delivering low oxygen concentrations
• Allows freedom of movement; doesn't interfere with eating or talking

Disadvantages
• Can't be used when patient has complete nasal obstruction; for example, mucosal edema or polyps
• May cause headaches or dry mucous membranes if flow rate exceeds 6 liters/minute
• Can dislodge easily
• Strap may pinch chin if adjusted too tightly.
• Patient must be alert and cooperative to keep cannula in place.

Nursing considerations
• Remove and clean the cannula with a wet cloth every 8 hours. Give good mouth and nose care.
• If the patient's restless, tape the cannula in place.
• Check for pressure areas under his nose and over his ears. Apply gauze padding, if necessary.
• Moisten the patient's lips and nose with water-soluble jelly, but take care not to occlude the cannula.

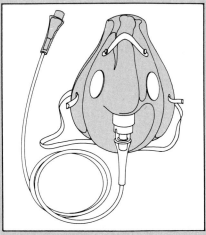

SIMPLE FACE MASK
(low-flow system)

Benefits
• Effectively delivers high oxygen concentrations
• Humidification can be increased by using large-bore tubing and aerosol mask.
• Doesn't dry mucous membranes

Disadvantages
• Hot and confining; may irritate skin
• Tight seal necessary for higher oxygen concentration may cause discomfort.
• Interferes with eating and talking
• Can't deliver less than 40% oxygen
• Impractical for long-term therapy

Nursing considerations
• Don't use on a patient with COPD.
• Place pads between the mask and bony facial parts.
• Periodically massage the patient's face with your fingertips.
• Wash and dry his face every 2 hours.
• For adequate flush, maintain a flow rate of 5 liters/minute.
• Don't adjust the strap too tightly.
• Remove and clean the mask with a wet cloth every 8 hours.

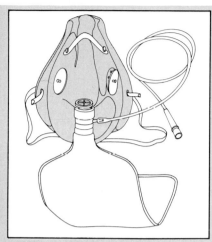

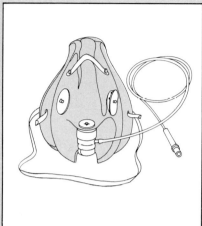

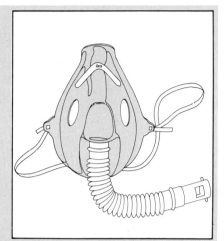

PARTIAL REBREATHING MASK
(low-flow system)

Benefits
• Oxygen reservoir bag lets patient rebreathe his exhaled air, which is high in oxygen content. This increases his fraction of inspired oxygen (FIO_2) concentration.
• Safety valve allows patient to inhale room air if oxygen source fails.
• Effectively delivers higher oxygen concentrations (35% to 60%)
• Easily humidifies oxygen
• Doesn't dry mucous membranes
• Most types easily converted to nonbreathing mask by inserting rubber flange over reservoir bag

Disadvantages
• Tight seal necessary to ensure accurate oxygen concentrations may cause discomfort.
• Interferes with eating and talking
• Hot and confining; may irritate skin
• Bag may twist or kink.
• Impractical for long-term use

Nursing considerations
• To initially fill the bag, apply the mask as the patient exhales.
• Never let the bag totally deflate during inhalation. Increase liter flow, if necessary, to avoid deflation.
• Avoid twisting the bag.
• Keep the mask snug to prevent inhalation of room air.

NONREBREATHING MASK
(low-flow system)

Benefits
• Delivers highest possible oxygen concentration (60% to 90%) short of intubation and mechanical ventilation
• Effective for short-term therapy
• Doesn't dry mucous membranes
• Can be converted to a partial rebreathing mask, if necessary.

Disadvantages
• Requires a tight seal, which may be hard to maintain; may cause discomfort
• May irritate skin
• Impractical for long-term therapy

Nursing considerations
• Never let the bag totally deflate during inhalation. Increase liter flow, if necessary, to avoid deflation.
• Avoid twisting the bag.
• Keep the mask snug to prevent inhalation of room air.
• Make sure all rubber flaps remain in place.
• Watch the patient closely for signs of oxygen toxicity.

VENTURI MASK
(high-flow system)

Benefits
• Delivers exact oxygen concentration despite patient's respiratory pattern
• Diluter jets can be changed or dial turned to change oxygen concentration.
• Doesn't dry mucous membranes
• Can be used to deliver humidity or aerosol therapy
• Delivers only prescribed oxygen concentration

Disadvantages
• Hot and confining; mask may irritate skin.
• FIO_2 concentration may be altered if mask doesn't fit snugly, if tubing's kinked, if oxygen intake ports are blocked, or if less-than-recommended liter flow is used.
• Interferes with eating and talking
• Condensation may collect and drain on patient when humidification's used.

Nursing considerations
• Check arterial blood gas measurements frequently.
• Soften the skin around the patient's mouth with petrolatum to prevent irritation.
• Remove and clean the mask with a wet cloth every 8 hours.

EMBOLISM MANAGEMENT CONTINUED

SURGERY: THE LAST RESORT

A patient with acute, massive PE may require surgery if he can't receive anticoagulant or fibrinolytic drugs, if he develops new emboli after treatment, or if he has chronic PE. Two surgical techniques are used: vena caval interruption and pulmonary embolectomy (which may include ligation).

The goal of vena caval interruption is to prevent migration of small, recurrent emboli by blocking their access route to the lungs. The surgeon can choose from two different methods. In the direct method, he fastens multichanneled clips inside the vena cava; the clips allow only partial blood flow. In the transvenous method, he passes a filtering device, such as a tiny umbrella, through a catheter threaded into the vein. The umbrella acts as a sieve to keep emboli from migrating upward to the lungs. Using fluoroscopy, some filters can be placed through the jugular vein, requiring only local anesthesia.

Pulmonary embolectomy involves extracting the embolus from the pulmonary arterial system. It's usually done only when a patient's in shock from severe massive pulmonary edema and not responding to other therapy. Some surgeons pass a catheter through the femoral vein to the right heart and into the pulmonary artery. Once the catheter tip's in place, suction is applied and the blockage is removed. This procedure can be performed while the patient's under local anesthesia.

However, in most cases, a thoracotomy is performed with the patient requiring general anesthesia and cardiopulmonary bypass. During this procedure, the surgeon may also ligate the inferior vena cava (in a woman, he may ligate the left ovarian vein as well). Unfortunately, ligation isn't a foolproof solution for PE prevention. In many cases, complete ligation results in the rapid development of collateral vessels— new passageways for the emboli to travel to the lungs.

Embolism surgery

A vena caval umbrella traps emboli while permitting blood flow to the lungs.

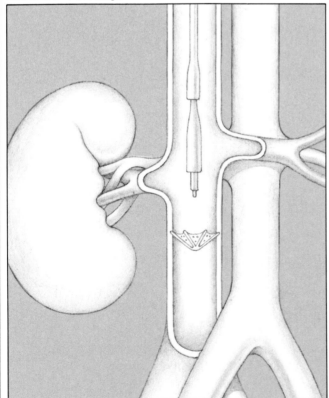

In vena caval ligation, the surgeon ties off the vena cava to stop small, recurrent emboli from migrating to the lungs.

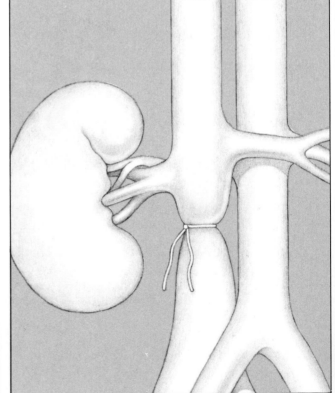

A.R.D.S.

CASE IN POINT

THE MERIT OF A SUSPICIOUS MIND

Marilyn Heron, a 77-year-old retired bank officer, is admitted to the medical/surgical unit with disseminated intravascular coagulation (DIC) resulting from gram-negative septicemia. You administer heparin I.V., as ordered, to control active bleeding.

When blood tests show her hemoglobin at 10.1 g/100 ml and hematocrit at 38%, you transfuse one unit of packed red blood cells, as ordered. However, Mrs. Heron then develops a transfusion reaction, which requires treatment with epinephrine and normal saline solution at a keep-vein-open rate. Her condition improves several hours later, and you breathe a sigh of relief.

The next day, her vital signs remain stable and she appears alert and oriented, although her respiratory rate's 30.

Later, however, the night nurse observes that Mrs. Heron's respiratory rate has increased and now fluctuates between 33 and 40. She also notes that the patient's becoming increasingly anxious and confused.

A day later, you find Mrs. Heron pale and confused. When you ask her where she is, she replies, "At my sister's house." Although she has no history of respiratory injury, you suspect her signs and symptoms may be caused by hypoxia—not by a reaction to hospitalization as you first thought. Your suspicions intensify when you notice bibasicular rales and rhonchi while auscultating. You notify the doctor, who orders arterial blood gas (ABG) testing.

The results confirm hypoxia: pH 7.5; $PaCO_2$ 27; PaO_2 46; SaO_2 79%; HCO_3^- 18. The doctor orders a portable chest X-ray and 40% O_2 by Venturi mask. At this point, Mrs. Heron's restless and dyspneic and must use her accessory chest muscles to breathe.

The next ABG measurements show Mrs. Heron hasn't responded to oxygen therapy. The doctor decides to intubate her and initiate ventilatory support. But when an increase in oxygen flow to 60% doesn't significantly increase her PaO_2, he determines that Mrs. Heron has probably developed adult respiratory distress syndrome (ARDS) secondary to DIC. He orders positive end-expiratory pressure (PEEP). Within an hour, her oxygenation improves.

After 6 days on PEEP, her ABG levels return to normal and her lungs clear.

Mrs. Heron could have become a mortality statistic: About 80% of ARDS patients die without early ventilatory support. But because you kept an open mind and used your assessment skills expertly, you detected suspicious findings early enough to give your patient a fighting chance for survival.

A DESTRUCTIVE CHAIN OF EVENTS

ARDS begins with shock or a shocklike state and leads to pulmonary hypoperfusion, edema, and atelectasis. The shock may result from an indirect injury such as sepsis, fluid overload, disseminated intravascular coagulation, or pancreatitis. But it can also be caused by direct injury such as near drowning, aspiration pneumonia, toxic chemical inhalation, or chest trauma.

First stage: Injury. Lung injury—either direct or indirect—reduces blood flow to the lungs, allowing platelets to aggregate in the alveolar capillaries. This leads to the formation of multiple microthrombi. The platelets also release serotonin, adenosine diphosphate, lysosomal enzymes, and histamine—substances that inflame and damage the respiratory membrane and make the capillary membrane abnormally permeable. Plasma and proteins leak from the capillaries into the interstitial spaces, alveoli, and small airways of the lungs (see illustration at right). The patient now has pulmonary edema.

CONTINUED ON PAGE 96

Capillary leakage

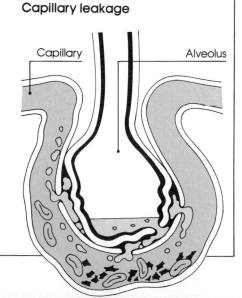

Capillary   Alveolus

A.R.D.S. CONTINUED

A DESTRUCTIVE CHAIN OF EVENTS CONTINUED

As pulmonary edema is developing, a process that will lead to atelectasis is also taking place. Hypoperfusion and edema damage Type II pneumocytes—cells that produce lung surfactant, the substance that helps prevent alveolar collapse. With decreased amounts of surfactant, alveoli collapse (see illustration below).

Collapsing alveolus

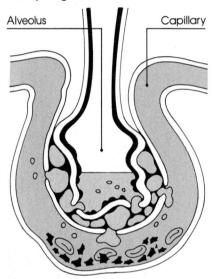

Alveolus   Capillary

Your patient now has alveoli that are either collapsed or filled with fluid—in other words, unavailable for gas exchange. Consequently, his lung compliance decreases and atelectasis develops.

Now the patient hyperventilates to try to take in more oxygen. But because carbon dioxide's more soluble than oxygen, it crosses the respiratory membrane more easily than oxygen and may be lost with each exhalation. The patient develops hypocapnia as carbon dioxide levels drop. Despite hyperventilation, hypoxia worsens. Alveolar inflammation leads to fibrosis, which further impairs gas exchange (see next illustration). Unless treated, hypoxia and metabolic acidosis may be fatal.

One condition, many names. ARDS isn't a clearly defined disease but a catchall term for a group of signs and symptoms. Only recently has ARDS become the agreed-upon term for the following conditions:
• shock lung syndrome
• wet lung
• Da Nang lung
• white lung
• stiff lung
• adult hyaline membrane disease
• respiratory lung
• acute ventilatory insufficiency
• post-pump lung
• acute pulmonary insufficiency
• post-traumatic pulmonary insufficiency
• noncardiogenic pulmonary edema
• hemorrhagic pulmonary edema.

Atelectatic alveolus

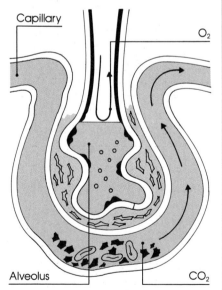

Capillary O_2

Alveolus CO_2

SIGNS AND SYMPTOMS

If you suspect your patient has ARDS, keep in mind that early signs and symptoms are subtle and may be easily overlooked or misinterpreted. And remember—although at first he may have an occasional cough or slight tachypnea, his breath sounds may be normal.

First-stage symptoms. In the first stage of ARDS (the 24 to 48 hours that ARDS usually takes to develop), your patient may become increasingly restless, irritable, and confused and may have difficulty concentrating. His pulse and temperature may be elevated. As mentioned earlier, he may cough occasionally and have slight tachypnea. Auscultation usually reveals clear lungs.

A growing distress. As hypoxia and hypocapnia progress, the patient's condition worsens. Dyspnea and diaphoresis become obvious. Expect increased confusion, tachypnea, and tachycardia, as well as grunting respirations with intercostal or suprasternal retraction. Now auscultation will reveal rhonchi, rales, and bronchial respirations. At this stage, cyanosis sets in. Consider refractory hypoxia—unresponsiveness to oxygen therapy, even at a high-flow rate—a telltale sign of ARDS.

As ARDS advances, the patient's condition deteriorates. He produces a thick, frothy, sticky sputum. Hypoxia worsens and respiratory distress intensifies. Arterial blood gas values will reveal decreasing $PaCO_2$ (respiratory alkalosis), decreasing HCO_3^- (metabolic acidosis), and falling PaO_2—despite oxygen therapy. In the end stage of ARDS, the patient can no longer compensate by hyperventilating and will experience respiratory acidosis from CO_2 retention.

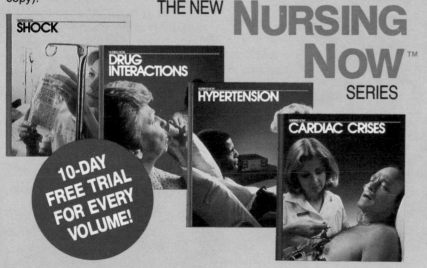
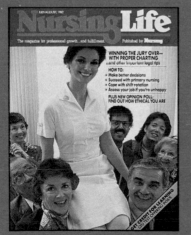

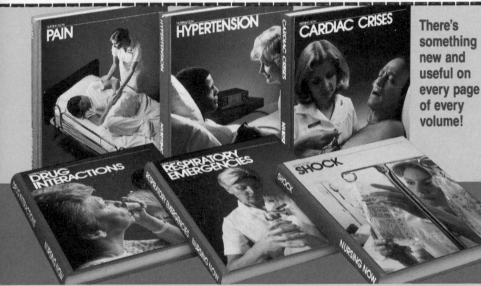

There's something new and useful on every page of every volume!

The series that keeps you up to date on the latest advances in nursing.

© 1984 Springhouse Corporation

DIAGNOSING A.R.D.S.

In addition to arterial blood gas measurements, the doctor may order these other diagnostic tests to determine the cause of ARDS:
• *Pulmonary artery catheterization.* This test determines pulmonary capillary wedge pressure, which can help identify the cause of pulmonary edema. During the procedure, the doctor can also collect a pulmonary arterial blood sample to determine tissue oxygen saturation.
• *Culture and sensitivity and Gram stain of sputum.* These help detect viral, bacterial, or fungal pneumonia.

• *Blood cultures.* These can detect septicemia.
• *Toxicology screen.* This test reveals drug ingestion.
• *Serum amylases determination.* This test can identify pancreatitis.
• *Chest X-rays.* In early ARDS, X-rays show bilateral diffuse infiltrates. X-rays taken in later stages show the lungs with a ground-glass appearance. Eventually, whiteouts appear in both fields.

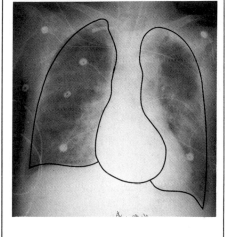

A.R.D.S. on X-ray
In this chest X-ray of a patient with ARDS, the lungs show characteristic whiteouts in both fields.

MANAGING A.R.D.S.

The goals of ARDS treatment are to increase PaO$_2$, PaCO$_2$, and tissue oxygenation; minimize oxygen consumption; and prevent or treat complications. Monitoring your patient's ABG values frequently will help you evaluate his progress.

Some ARDS patients may benefit from ventilatory assistance with continuous positive airway pressure (CPAP). If your patient's hypoxia doesn't respond to CPAP, he'll require intubation, volume ventilation, and positive end-expiratory pressure (PEEP). Other supportive measures include fluid monitoring, diuretics, and correction of electrolyte and acid-base abnormalities.

CPAP. When a patient can't maintain PaO$_2$ above 50 mm Hg when receiving oxygen at 50% concentration—but *can* breathe on his own—the doctor will probably order CPAP to ensure continuous positive pressure to the alveoli even after expiration. CPAP is usually delivered through a tight-fitting mask.

When administering CPAP, gradually increase the pressure in increments of 2 to 5 cm by

adding water to the water chamber until it reaches the prescribed level. In most cases, 10 cmH$_2$O keeps the patient adequately oxygenated when he's receiving an oxygen concentration of 50% or less.

If effective, CPAP will improve arterial oxygenation, increase functional residual capacity (the amount of air remaining in the patient's lungs after a normal expiration), and increase lung compliance.

PEEP. If your patient *can't* breathe on his own and can't maintain PaO$_2$ above 50 mm Hg at 50% oxygen concentration, he'll need PEEP. By keeping the alveoli open longer, PEEP increases PaO$_2$ without raising oxygen concentration. Increasing PaO$_2$ by using a higher oxygen concentration, you'll remember, can cause serious side effects.

To ensure optimal PEEP effectiveness, the ventilator must control respiration completely. For this reason, the doctor may order a skeletal muscle relaxant, a tranquilizer, or both, to prevent the patient's natural inspiratory effort from interfering with preset PEEP pressure.

Like CPAP, PEEP improves arterial oxygenation and functional residual capacity and increases lung compliance. However, the patient on PEEP risks barotrauma, impaired cardiac output, and other complications associated with mechanical ventilation. To minimize these risks, the doctor may order lower PEEP levels (if possible) or blood products to expand intravascular volume.

Pulmonary artery catheterization. Monitoring fluid pressure with pulmonary capillary wedge pressure (PCWP) can help your patient maintain balanced perfusion—an essential step in ARDS management. Fluid overload may worsen pulmonary edema, in turn increasing intrapulmonary shunting and further decreasing lung compliance. On the other hand, underhydration may further impair perfusion—already compromised by ARDS.

To obtain PCWP, a balloon-tipped, flow-directed catheter is threaded to the junction of the heart's vena cava and right atrium. When the doctor inflates the balloon, venous circulation

CONTINUED ON PAGE 98

A.R.D.S. CONTINUED

MANAGING A.R.D.S.
CONTINUED

carries the catheter tip through the right atrium and ventricle to a pulmonary artery branch, where the balloon wedges itself.

Once it's wedged, you'll need to get a pressure reading. If your patient's PCWP is higher than 12 mm Hg, suspect overhydration; if it's under 6 mm Hg, suspect underhydration.

Other supportive measures. Additional ARDS treatments are aimed at controlling sepsis, fever, agitation, and physical activity—conditions that increase oxygen consumption. Antipyretics, tepid baths, and a hypothermia blanket may be ordered to treat fever. Sedatives such as haloperidol, diazepam, and morphine help reduce agitation and physical activity. Morphine also helps slow the patient's respiratory rate, which may be 45 or higher in ARDS. If your patient's receiving morphine, keep naloxone handy to reverse side effects such as hypotension or ileus.

Special Note:

Many disorders can lead to ARDS. By identifying patients at risk, you can help prevent ARDS from developing. Check closely for even minor changes in respiratory rate, vital capacity, and blood gas values in any patient with one of the following disorders: shock of any type, infection, toxic chemical inhalation (including oxygen at high concentrations), hematologic or metabolic disorders, drug overdose, liquid aspiration, or trauma.

COMPARING VENTILATORS

Ventilators come in two main types—volume-cycled and pressure-cycled—which end inspiration after delivery of a preset volume or pressure. A third ventilator type is time-cycled, meaning it ends inspiration after a preset time has elapsed. (The high-frequency jet ventilator's an example.) Use the chart below to compare ventilators.

VOLUME-CYCLED VENTILATOR

Features
• Ventilator delivers preset tidal volume to lungs.
• Inspiration ends with preset volume delivery.
• Amount of pressure delivered varies with patient's lung compliance.
• Preset volume determines inspiration depth.
• Pop-off safety valve releases pressure when high pressure's required to deliver preset volume.
• Oxygen concentration can be varied between 21% and 100% by changing oxygen flow rate.
• Automatic sigh mechanism helps prevent atelectasis.
• Alarms indicate problems with volume and pressure delivery and sensitivity.
• Electricity powers ventilator.

Indications
• Long-term ventilation
• Severe bronchospasm or adult respiratory distress syndrome (ARDS), which require inflation pressures greater than 40 cmH$_2$O
• Flail chest, when stabilization requires adequate lung expansion
• Pulmonary edema with decreased compliance
• Cardiac or respiratory arrest
• Central nervous system (CNS) and musculoskeletal disorders (for example, Guillain-Barré syndrome)
• Complex thoracic surgery

• Exacerbated chronic lung disease
• Crushed chest injuries
• PEEP therapy

Advantages
• Changes in airway resistance or compliance have little effect on volume delivered.
• Ventilator delivers precise oxygen concentration.
• Ventilator provides automatic sighing.

Disadvantages
None

PRESSURE-CYCLED VENTILATOR

Features
• Ventilator delivers preset pressure to patient's lungs.
• Inspiration ends with preset pressure delivery.
• Volume of air delivered varies with patient's lung compliance.
• Preset pressure determines inspiration depth.
• Air-mix dial delivers oxygen concentration between 40% and 90%; wall outlet delivers 100% oxygen; compressed air from wall outlet delivers 21% oxygen; blenders of compressed air and oxygen deliver oxygen concentrations ranging from 21% to 90%.
• Sigh mechanism operates manually.
• Oxygen or compressed air powers ventilator.

Indications
• Short-term ventilation (for example, during postoperative recovery, acute lung disease, drug overdose, or acute airway obstruction)
• Neuromuscular disease such as myasthenia gravis
• Neurologic disorders, such as head trauma, that damage respi-

ratory centers in the brain but don't affect lungs
• Intermittent positive pressure breathing (IPPB) therapy

Advantages
• Pressure cycling may ventilate obstructed air passages more efficiently than volume cycling.

Disadvantages
• Older models have limited flow-rate and inspiratory pressure options.
• Rapid cycling (shortened inspiratory time), caused by a kink in tubing or an obstruction from fluid

or secretions, often occurs.
• Continuation of inspiratory phase (a malfunction caused by leaks or electrical disconnection) often occurs.
• A decrease in lung compliance requires a pressure adjustment to maintain alveolar ventilation.
• Routine care, such as turning and suctioning, and coughing and deep-breathing exercises may reduce tidal volume.
• The pressure-cycled ventilator may not deliver minute volumes necessary for long-term mechanical ventilation, since lung compliance changes can alter the tidal volume delivered.

Advantages
• May decrease time required on ventilator and shorten weaning period
• Achieves alveolar ventilation without generating high-peak inspiratory pressure
• Prevents loss of tidal volume through airway disruption site by delivering constant pressure
• Provides lower CO_2 clearance and higher $PaCO_2$
• Decreases risk of barotrauma

Disadvantage
• Long-term effects unknown

Volume-cycled ventilator

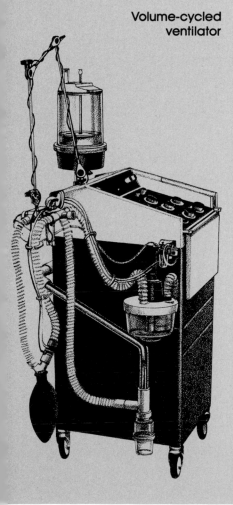

HIGH–FREQUENCY JET VENTILATOR (time-cycled)

Features
• Ventilator delivers 100 to 600 breaths/minute with low tidal volume under considerable pressure.
• Jet flow transfers kinetic energy to gases in upper airway moving in the direction of jet flow.
• Inspiration ends after a preset timing cycle has elapsed.
• Timer allows selection of respiratory rate and inspiratory/expiratory pressure.
• Jet mixing supplies air and oxygen at a pressure of 50 psi.
• Alarm sounds when system malfunctions.
• Driving pressure determines tidal volume.

Indications
• Bronchopleural fistula
• Tracheoesophageal fistula
• Barotrauma, such as pneumothorax and pneumomediastinum
• Low pulmonary compliance (experimentally)
• ARDS (experimentally)
• PEEP therapy (experimentally)
• Flail chest or thoracic trauma

Pressure-cycled ventilator

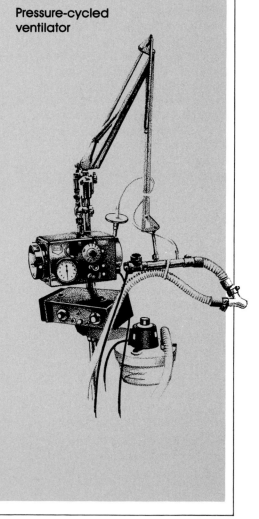

A.R.D.S. CONTINUED

HIGH-FREQUENCY JET VENTILATION

A new mechanical ventilation technique may be more efficient and safer than traditional systems for patients with acute respiratory failure, particularly those with ARDS. Called high-frequency jet ventilation (HFJV), this experimental technique may eventually become widely accepted.

Old versus new. Like pressure-cycled and volume-cycled ventilators, HFJV ventilates the alveoli. What makes HFJV potentially superior to traditional ventilators is the method by which it supplies air and oxygen to the lungs. Small pulsed jets of gas enter the airway at high respiratory rates (usually 100 to 600 breaths/minute) through a small catheter or an extra lumen in an endotracheal tube. (HFJV can also be delivered through a transtracheal catheter, eliminating the need for endotracheal intubation or tracheostomy.)

Because of its small tidal volume and fast respiratory rates, HFJV keeps airway pressure low and produces only minimal alveolar distention, thus stabilizing alveolar ventilation. It also minimizes the risks of barotrauma and hemodynamic compromise. Some researchers suggest cardiac output may be greater with HFJV than with traditional ventilators, because its lower airway pressures interfere less with venous return to the heart. According to one theory, cardiac output may increase if HFJV is synchronized with the patient's heart rate.

Nursing considerations. Ensuring adequate airway humidification is your major priority when caring for a patient on HFJV. To guard against the ventilator's drying effect, monitor the water level and function of the cascade humidifier.

You may also need to suction your patient to prevent airway obstruction. When necessary, hyperoxygenate him first; then suction rapidly. Notify the doctor immediately if secretions are scant or viscous. He may order a mucolytic agent or ask you to irrigate the airway with 5 to 10 ml of sterile normal saline solution before suctioning.

If the jet ventilator's supplying all the patient's ventilatory needs, he won't produce breath sounds. If the patient's taking spontaneous breaths along with the ventilator—as many patients do—breath sounds can be auscultated.

Also, observe the patient carefully for the following signs and symptoms of barotrauma: dyspnea, decreased or absent breath sounds, restlessness, pain, abnormal chest-wall motion, tracheal shift, hyperresonance to percussion, crepitus, and hypoxia. Notify the doctor at once if any of these indications occur.

Any patient on a ventilator may be anxious about the procedure. Remember to provide emotional support.

Note: If your patient's using an experimental high-frequency jet ventilator, make sure he or a family member consents to HFJV therapy.

CARING FOR A PATIENT ON PANCURONIUM THERAPY

Ventilating the patient with ARDS is never easy because the disorder stiffens the lungs, reducing lung compliance. High-peak ventilatory pressure needed to increase PaO_2 may limit the patient's ventilation and increase the risk of complications. To prevent these problems, the doctor may order pancuronium (Pavulon), a neuromuscular blocking agent. By inducing complete skeletal muscle relaxation while maintaining a fully alert central nervous system, pancuronium improves the patient's response to mechanical ventilation.

Pancuronium induces paralysis in less than 3 minutes. The doctor will probably order an initial dose of 4 to 8 mg, administered I.V., then 2 to 8 mg in 30- to 90-minute intervals.

When administering this potent drug, follow these special guidelines:
• Explain the drug's effects to the patient and his family. Reassure and reorient the patient frequently during therapy.
• Administer a sedative, as ordered, to diminish the patient's perception and recall of paralysis.
• Make sure ventilator connections are tight at all times.
• To prevent corneal abrasions, tape the patient's eyes shut. Remove the tape every 2 to 4 hours and instill artificial tears.
• Monitor his fluid intake and output (renal dysfunction may prolong the drug's duration of action).
• Closely monitor his heart and respiratory rates.
• Check electrolyte levels regularly and compare them with baseline measurements (an electrolyte imbalance may increase pancuronium's neuromuscular effects).

NEAR DROWNING

DEFINING THE EMERGENCY

Drowning, the fourth leading cause of accidental death, claims about 8,000 American lives each year. Children under age 4 account for nearly half of these deaths. Many drowning and near-drowning victims find themselves in water unexpectedly; for example, after a boating accident or a fall from a dock or bridge. Other victims are swimmers who can't stay afloat—for reasons that range from poor swimming skills and fatigue to a medical emergency such as myocardial infarction.

You may be surprised to learn that the drowning victim doesn't die from water aspiration but from hypoxia caused by asphyxiation. The near-drowning victim, who by definition survives the accident, also becomes hypoxic.

Chain of events. Consider the chain of events leading to drowning or near drowning: While submerged, the victim swallows or aspirates water. In response, he holds his breath, which increases his arterial carbon dioxide level. After a certain point, however, increased carbon dioxide levels stimulate the brain's respiratory center, forcing the victim to breathe.

However, as he breathes, he swallows or aspirates greater quantities of water, causing him to vomit and perhaps aspirate some vomitus. He then loses consciousness, convulses, and aspirates more water. This type of drowning, called *wet drowning*, is the most common drowning type.

In *dry drowning*, the first aspiration causes laryngospasm, which blocks the trachea and prevents further aspiration. The victim asphyxiates, becomes hypoxic, and loses consciousness. The dry-drowning victim has a better chance of surviving.

A third drowning type, *secondary drowning*, can occur several minutes or even several days after the accident if respiratory distress (for example, aspiration pneumonia or pulmonary edema) recurs.

SALTWATER AND FRESHWATER ASPIRATION: TWO ROUTES TO HYPOXIA

Although the cause of death in drowning—and the ultimate danger in near drowning—is hypoxia, the type of fluid aspirated determines how hypoxia develops. Fresh water, which is hypotonic compared to blood, rapidly penetrates the pulmonary capillary membrane. Large amounts of lung surfactant are either lost or altered, causing alveolar collapse, intrapulmonary shunting, and hypoxia.

Salt water, which is hypertonic compared to blood, disrupts osmotic pressure, forcing fluid into the alveoli. Pulmonary edema, intrapulmonary shunting, and hypoxia result.

The chart on the next page shows how fluid aspiration affects the body.

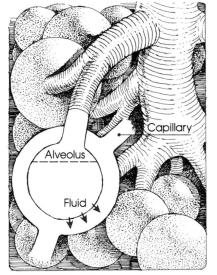

Freshwater aspiration
When a hypotonic fluid such as fresh water enters the alveolus, it can chemically alter the capillary membrane and destroy pulmonary surfactant. Intrapulmonary shunting and hypoxia result. The fresh water also passes through the alveolar membrane and causes hemodilution, as shown in the illustration above. This sudden circulatory overload is thought to cause freshwater pulmonary edema. In rare cases, ventricular fibrillation and death result.

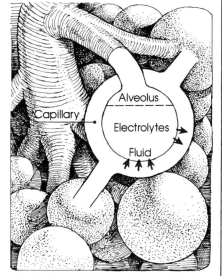

Saltwater aspiration
Salt water's hypertonicity draws fluid from the pulmonary capillary bed into the pulmonary interstitium and the alveoli (see the illustration above). Consequently, the lung parenchyma undergoes damage. Fluid floods the alveoli, leading to intrapulmonary shunting and hypoxia.

NEAR DROWNING CONTINUED

HOW FLUID ASPIRATION AFFECTS VARIOUS BODY SYSTEMS AND INDEXES

ARTERIAL BLOOD GASES

Effect
Hypoxia

BLOOD VOLUME

Effect
Salt water: Persistent hypovolemia from hypertonic fluid entering the alveoli
Fresh water: Transient hypervolemia from rapid absorption of hypotonic fluid into the circulation

CARDIAC EFFECTS

Effect
Ventricular fibrillation from aspiration of large amounts of fluid (rare)

HEMOGLOBIN

Effect
Possible hemoglobin decrease; hemolysis after aspiration of 0.11 ml of fluid/kg of body weight

NEUROLOGIC EFFECTS

Effect
Altered mental status or coma from cerebral anoxia

SERUM ELECTROLYTES

Effect
Changes usually insignificant; severe hypoxia and acidosis may cause hyperkalemia

URINARY EFFECTS

Effect
Acute renal failure from hypotension and hypoxia

NEAR DROWNING SIGNS AND SYMPTOMS

Immediately after a near drowning, your first priority is to check the victim for the following signs and symptoms of asphyxia and pulmonary edema:
• rapidly worsening dyspnea
• apnea
• wheezing, rales, and rhonchi
• productive cough with pink, frothy sputum
• substernal chest pain that worsens with breathing
• tachycardia
• vomiting
• abdominal distention
• cyanosis
• confusion
• lethargy
• irritability
• restlessness
• unconsciousness
• seizure
• coma
• elevated body temperature. (However, if the accident occurred in cold water, the patient's temperature may be abnormally low).
• respiratory or cardiac arrest.

"Both saltwater and freshwater aspiration can cause fluid overload or depletion. Make sure you carefully evaluate the fluid status of any near-drowning victim."

Paul C. Summerell, RN, BSN
Assistant head nurse
Medical Intensive Care Unit
Duke University Medical Center
Durham, N.C.

HELPING THE NEAR–DROWNING VICTIM

You can begin cardiopulmonary resuscitation (CPR) as soon as the victim's head is above water. (Since most drowning victims die from lack of air, not water aspiration, it's not necessary to drain water from the victim's lungs or stomach). If you suspect a spinal injury, place a board under the victim's head and back while he's still in the water.

When the victim arrives at the hospital, your first priority is to maintain an open airway. Continue CPR, if necessary. Then take the following measures:
• Relieve hypoxia. Administer low-percentage oxygen until you can obtain ABG measurements. Then ventilate the patient, as ordered, using intermittent positive pressure breathing (IPPB) with 100% oxygen or positive end-expiratory pressure (PEEP). Suction the patient's airway frequently to remove secretions.
• Monitor vital signs. Continue to do this even after the patient's condition has stabilized. Check his central venous pressure to assess cardiopulmonary status. Stay alert for signs of secondary drowning and increased respiratory distress (for example, confusion, chest pain, and adventitious breath sounds).
• Relieve abdominal distention. Insert a nasogastric tube and connect it to suction, as ordered.
• Administer appropriate medications. Be prepared to give isoproterenol to relieve bronchospasm; steroids to stabilize damaged capillary walls; and antibiotics to prevent infection.
• Monitor the patient's intake and output. Insert an indwelling (Foley) catheter and start an I.V. line to administer plasma.

TOXIC CHEMICAL INHALATION

THE ROUTE TO RESPIRATORY DISTRESS

As the use of synthetic materials increases, so does the risk of a chemical accident leading to toxic lung injury—a dangerous respiratory disorder resulting from toxic chemical inhalation. Workers or bystanders may suffer toxic chemical inhalation from an accident, such as a fire at a chemical plant or an explosion at an oil refinery.

Toxic lung injury can occur within minutes after exposure to noxious chemicals contained in smoke or gas. Without proper treatment, this injury can lead to respiratory failure.

Smoke vs. gas inhalation. How a person responds to a certain toxic chemical depends on whether he's inhaled it in the form of smoke or gas. Initial responses to smoke inhalation include bronchiolar constriction, laryngeal edema, and increased carboxyhemoglobin levels. Cough, stridor, and cherry red mucosa are early signs and symptoms. The victim may also suffer delayed responses, such as increased pulmonary capillary permeability and destruction of lung parenchyma. Late signs and symptoms include dyspnea, rales, rhonchi, increased sputum production, and lung hyperinflation.

Responses to gas inhalation vary according to gas solubility. A person who's inhaled a water-soluble gas such as ammonia usually flees the area immediately because this gas type is extremely irritating to the upper airways. By fleeing, he reduces the risk of lung damage.

But if he's trapped in the contaminated area, he'll inhale a much greater volume of gas. Consequently, the gas penetrates deeper into the respiratory system, causing potentially acute respiratory dysfunction.

Insoluble gases such as nitrogen dioxide cause only mild upper airway irritation. A person exposed to such a gas is more likely to inhale a greater volume of gas before fleeing and thus suffer greater lung damage at the alveolar level.

IDENTIFYING RISK FACTORS

Certain patients are more likely than others to sustain significant lung damage from toxic chemical inhalation. The following factors predispose a patient to serious lung damage:

• *Preexisting lung disease* that reduces ventilation, disturbs cell function, or destroys lung tissue; for example, tuberculosis, chronic obstructive pulmonary disease (COPD), or pleurisy. (Pulmonary edema is an exception. The excess fluid this condition produces helps mobilize harmful particles before they can irritate the alveolar wall.)

• *Cigarette smoking* paralyzes the mucociliary escalator—a system in which the cilia and a mucous blanket propel airway particles upward. This leads to bronchoconstriction and thick mucous buildup, which compromise the lungs' normal defense mechanisms by impairing macrophagic activity.

• *Long-term exposure to toxic chemicals* can wear out the lungs' defense mechanisms. (Most lung diseases take years to develop.)

• *Exposure to high concentrations of toxic chemicals,* even over a short period of time, may overwhelm the lungs' defense mechanisms.

• *The size of a chemical's particles* determines where those particles lodge in the lungs. For example, particles 3 to 5 microns in diameter lodge in the alveoli and cause the greatest amount of damage. Particles less than 1 micron in diameter (for example, those in smoke, fumes, or aerosols) cause less serious injury, since they penetrate the alveolar walls and enter interstitial tissue.

Pulmonary edema and smoke inhalation

Pulmonary edema develops as damage to the capillary's endothelial layer increases pulmonary capillary permeability. This permits fluid to escape from the capillary, as shown close-up in the illustration below.

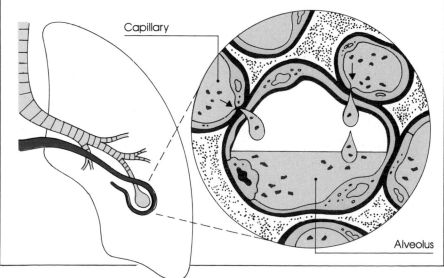

Capillary

Alveolus

TOXIC CHEMICAL INHALATION

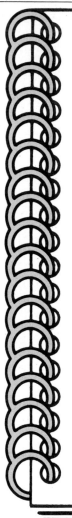

CRITICAL QUESTIONS

ASSESSING FOR TOXIC CHEMICAL INHALATION

Do you suspect your patient's respiratory crisis was caused by toxic chemical inhalation? Use this checklist as an assessment guide. If you can answer yes to all or most of these questions, chances are he's inhaled a toxic chemical.
• Did the accident occur in a confined area? How long did the patient remain in the area?
• During the accident, did any synthetic materials burn? If so, which material was it? How much? (The patient may not know the answers to these questions.)
• Does he complain of a burning pain in his chest or throat?
• Are his upper airways mildly irritated?
• Are his nasal hairs singed?
• Does he have any facial burns?
• Is he restless or agitated?
• Do you detect rales or rhonchi on auscultation?
• Is he dyspneic?
• Is he wheezing, coughing, or hoarse?
• Is he hypoxic?
• Does his sputum contain black carbon particles?

EMERGENCY CARE FOR TOXIC CHEMICAL INHALATION

Take these nursing steps immediately if your patient's suffering toxic chemical inhalation:
• Assess and maintain his airway, breathing, and circulation. Initiate cardiopulmonary resuscitation if necessary.
• Administer low-percentage humidified oxygen until you can obtain ABG measurements.
• Assist with insertion of an endotracheal tube to improve breathing.
• As ordered, ventilate the patient using IPPB with 100% oxygen to enhance inspired oxygen and blood distribution and improve the patient's ventilation/perfusion balance.
• Administer bronchodilators, as ordered, to help maintain airway patency.
• Give corticosteroids, if ordered, to help reduce tissue damage.
• Insert a nasogastric tube to help remove ingested chemicals.

Later, after the patient's condition has stabilized, teach him to perform postural drainage and encourage him to cough and deep breathe to help loosen and clear airway secretions.

COMBATING CARBON MONOXIDE POISONING

Carbon monoxide poisoning, one of the most common poisoning types, accompanies most inhalation injuries. Colorless, odorless, and tasteless, carbon monoxide is found in acetylene gas, automobile exhaust, carbonyl iron, coal gas, furnace gas, illuminating gas, and marsh gas.

Assessment. To assess the severity of carbon monoxide poisoning, the doctor will order blood tests to determine the patient's carboxyhemoglobin level. Signs and symptoms of carbon monoxide poisoning vary in severity depending on the carboxyhemoglobin level. A level of 20% causes headache and mild dyspnea, whereas a level between 20% and 40% produces fatigue, irritability, diminished judgment, dimmed vision, and nausea.

When the carboxyhemoglobin level's between 40% and 60%, the patient suffers confusion, hallucinations, ataxia, collapse, and coma. His skin and mucous membranes turn cherry red.

Although ABG measurements may reveal a normal PaO_2 level, oxygen release to peripheral tissues drops sharply when carboxyhemoglobin levels are high.

Management. The doctor will order 100% high-flow oxygen, which reduces the half-life of carboxyhemoglobin from 4 hours to 30 minutes. He may order blood transfusions or hyperbaric oxygen therapy. This treatment provides 100% oxygen at high pressure in a controlled environment.

In addition to administering oxygen, keep the patient on total bed rest for at least 48 hours, or as ordered. Also watch for signs and symptoms of reduced cardiac output or central nervous system impairment, which may not appear until 3 weeks later.

CHEST TRAUMA

CHEST TRAUMA BASICS

CHEST CONTUSION

FRACTURES

PNEUMOTHORAX

HEMOTHORAX

PENETRATING WOUNDS

CHEST TRAUMA BASICS

REVIEWING THE FACTS

Chest injuries—both blunt and penetrating—account for up to 75% of all trauma deaths in the United States. These injuries may damage the ribs, lungs, and major blood vessels, causing shock and massive internal or external hemorrhage. However, because of prompt assessment and expert medical care, nearly 60% of chest trauma victims now survive.

Blunt chest injuries—the aftermath of almost 25% of all automobile accidents—include pulmonary contusion, myocardial contusion, and rib or sternal fractures (simple, multiple, displaced, or jagged). These injuries can cause interstitial hemorrhage, edema, pulmonary lacerations, and bronchiolar rupture.

A penetrating chest wound, usually resulting from a gunshot or stab, causes lacerations and rapid blood loss. Depending on the weapon used, such a wound may damage bones, soft tissue, blood vessels, and nerves.

Complications. An extrathoracic chest injury such as a rib, sternum, or scapula fracture can lead to any of the following common intrathoracic injuries:
• pulmonary contusion
• myocardial contusion
• pneumothorax
• hemothorax
• hemopneumothorax
• cardiac tamponade
• ruptured aorta
• ruptured diaphragm.

ASSESSING THE INJURY

When checking a patient for chest injuries, try to determine exactly which chest area's involved. If the patient's conscious, ask him to show you where it hurts. Then, using your knowledge of thoracic anatomy, estimate which structures or blood vessels may have been damaged.

For example, the scapula usually reaches the level of the 7th rib posteriorly. The left ventricle is medial to the nipple line anteriorly. Surrounding the clavicle are the subclavian vessels, with the lungs' apices situated above them bilaterally. If any of these structures is displaced, suspect an injury in that region.

Injuries at the base of the neck may cause pneumothorax. Injuries at the nipple line may cause pulmonary or myocardial contusion; injuries between the 9th and 11th ribs may cause splenic rupture.

Study the information below to familiarize yourself with signs and symptoms of some common chest injuries:

Costochondral or chondrosternal separation, or costovertebral dislocation. Suspect it if the patient has a history of direct anterior impact to the chest, localized tenderness on palpation, and a clicking sensation during respiration.

Esophageal injury. Suspect it if the patient has cyanosis, dyspnea, upper abdominal pain, hypotension, subcutaneous emphysema in cervical or anterior thoracic regions, or signs and symptoms similar to tracheobronchial disruption that can't be attributed to tracheobronchial injury.

Hemothorax (torn blood vessels). Suspect it if the patient has hypotension, respiratory distress, tightness in the chest, signs of shock with severe bleeding, mediastinal shift on X-ray, and his-

tory of recent blunt chest trauma.

Injury to the heart or major cardiopulmonary vessels. Suspect it if the patient has ecchymotic areas over the chest wall, cardiac dysrhythmia, palpitations or precordial pain, cough, nausea, and vomiting.

Multiple rib fractures (flail chest). Suspect it if the patient has pain at the fracture site, subcutaneous chest movement, tenderness on palpation, bone crepitus, paradoxical chest movement, and breathing difficulty.

Penetrating or puncture wounds. Suspect it if the patient has subcutaneous emphysema, sucking sounds during respiration, visible lung through puncture, and signs of severe respiratory distress.

Rib fracture. Suspect it if the patient has localized tenderness or subcutaneous emphysema over the injured site, painful, difficult respirations, and paradoxical chest movement.

Sternal or chondral fracture. Suspect it if the patient has had a recent, severe chest-wall trauma; sharp, excruciating pain at the fracture site; swelling and visible deformity over the fracture site; subcutaneous emphysema; and tenderness when the sternum is palpated.

Tracheobronchial trauma. Suspect it if the patient has dyspnea, hemoptysis, cyanosis, and subcutaneous emphysema.

Trauma to pleura and/or lung (for example, lung contusion or pneumothorax). Suspect it if the patient complains of chest pain or shortness of breath, if you hear distant or absent breath sounds over the injured area, and if the patient has had a recent blunt chest injury.

Common chest injuries

This illustration shows the chest injuries you'll most frequently encounter.

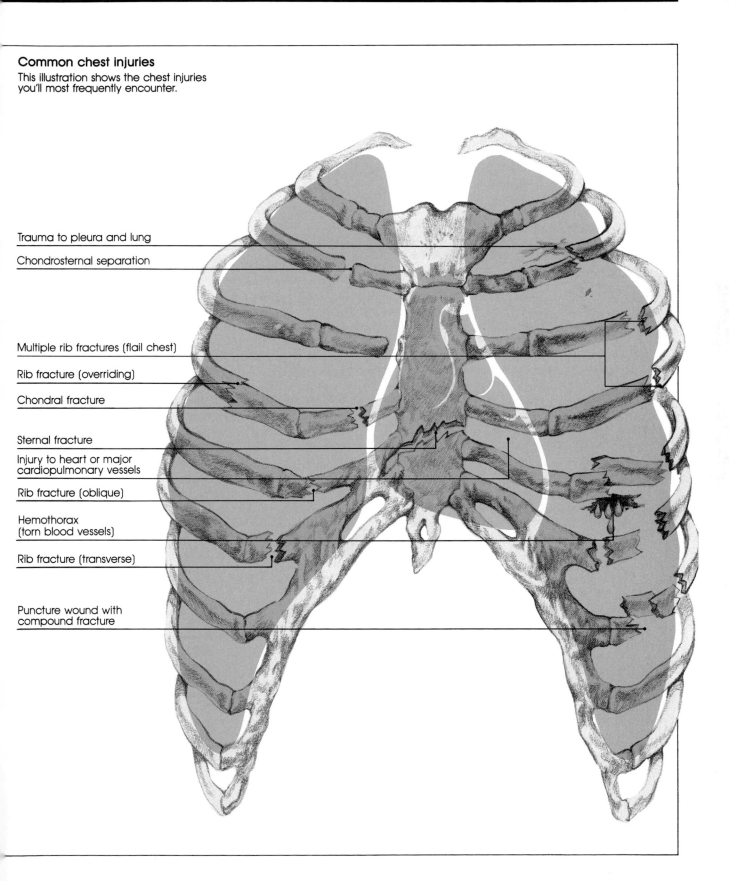

Trauma to pleura and lung

Chondrosternal separation

Multiple rib fractures (flail chest)

Rib fracture (overriding)

Chondral fracture

Sternal fracture

Injury to heart or major cardiopulmonary vessels

Rib fracture (oblique)

Hemothorax (torn blood vessels)

Rib fracture (transverse)

Puncture wound with compound fracture

CHEST TRAUMA BASICS CONTINUED

EVERY MINUTE COUNTS

When confronted with a chest trauma victim, you'll need to shift your normal nursing priorities. Don't waste time taking his history or performing a brief physical exam. Assess his condition rapidly, then take immediate steps to manage the wound.

First things first. Even if your patient's bleeding or in shock, your first priority is providing an open airway. If the patient's conscious, you may need to insert a nasopharyngeal airway to maintain patency. Insert a pharyngeal airway if the patient's unconscious. (If both pulse and airflow are absent, call for help and initiate cardiopulmonary resuscitation at once.)

Cervical spine precautions. Always assume a chest trauma victim has a cervical spine injury until X-rays prove otherwise. Initiate the following cervical spine precautions (unless a paramedic at the injury scene has done so already): Apply a cervical collar to immobilize his neck; then place him on a full-length backboard with sandbags secured on either side of his neck to prevent head movement. Check his level of consciousness.

Assessing the wound. When you're sure the patient's airway is open and he's breathing adequately, remove his clothing (cutting, if necessary) and examine his back and chest for lacerations and bruises. Also listen closely. If he has a sucking wound, you may hear it before you see it.

To care for a sucking chest wound, ask the patient to exhale with maximum force to expel air and fluid through the wound opening.

Close the wound quickly with a petrolatum gauze bandage, taping only three sides. To facilitate ventilation, keep the patient in high Fowler's position.

The overall picture. Evaluate your patient's skin color and temperature. Pale, cool, clammy skin may be an early sign of hypovolemic shock. Also check respiration depth, and compare length of inspirations and expirations. Is the patient using his accessory muscles to breathe? Check the position of his trachea. If it's shifted to one side, suspect tension pneumothorax or hemothorax.

Checking for bleeding. Note the color and consistency of bleeding and estimate the amount of blood loss. Don't forget to look beneath the patient when estimating blood loss to check for lacerated large blood vessels in the neck and thorax. If you find a cervical vessel laceration, consider your patient at serious risk of exsanguination. Immediately apply direct pressure to control bleeding, and ask a colleague to insert a nasopharyngeal or oropharyngeal airway to ensure patency. Then notify the doctor.

Assessing for rib fractures. Watch for paradoxical chest movement and other signs of broken ribs. For example, you may be able to feel the fracture, or you'll note swelling or crepitus over the fracture site. Your patient may tell you that he feels like holding or splinting the site.

Arranging for laboratory tests. Obtain a stat order for arterial blood gas measurements, complete blood count, and type and cross matching, as indicated.

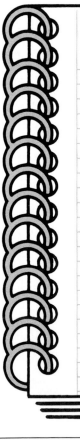

CRITICAL QUESTIONS

TAKING THE HISTORY

If your chest trauma patient's conscious and not suffering from severe dyspnea, ask him to describe the accident. This will help you focus your history-taking efforts. Here are some questions you may want to ask:

• How did the accident happen?

• If it involved an automobile, were you wearing a seatbelt?

• For a penetrating injury, what was the penetrating object? In the case of gunshot, what was the gun's caliber? If the patient doesn't know, check with the police or witnesses, if any.

• Where is your chest injured? Is that also where the pain's located?

• Describe the pain. Is it constant or intermittent? Does anything relieve it? Does anything make it worse? Does the pain occur when you breathe normally or only when you breathe deeply? Does holding the painful area relieve the pain? (Keep in mind that because the lungs have no pain-sensitive nerves, chest trauma pain's usually musculoskeletal.)

DIFFERENTIATING INTERSTITIAL FROM INTRAPLEURAL BLEEDING

When assessing a patient with chest trauma, make sure you check the color, consistency, and source of his bleeding. This will help you identify and manage the underlying cause. To help differentiate interstitial from intrapleural bleeding, follow these guidelines:

INTERSTITIAL BLEEDING

Color
Bright red
Flow
Pulsatile and rapid
Possible causes
• Rib fracture
• Internal soft tissue injuries
• Arterial lacerations from penetrating chest wound
Nursing actions
Apply direct pressure to control bleeding. If you see a laceration of the main hilar blood vessels, notify the doctor at once and prepare the patient for surgery.

INTRAPULMONARY BLEEDING

Color
Dark red
Flow
Slow and steady (may appear pulsatile if the patient's grunting on expiration)
Possible causes
• Pulmonary contusion
• Lung laceration from penetrating chest wound
• Sucking chest wound
Nursing actions
Apply direct pressure to control bleeding. Prepare the patient for surgery if you can't control pleurocutaneous bleeding, or if you detect intrapleural effusion or massive air leaks (from a bronchial rupture).

CHECKING FOR HYPOVOLEMIC SHOCK

Your chest trauma patient's skin is cool and clammy. He's restless and slightly tachypneic. You realize that these nonspecific symptoms may be caused by the transient stress of injury. But you should be concerned that hypovolemic shock may be the cause. This condition, which follows massive blood loss, may lead to irreversible cerebral and renal damage, cardiac arrest, and death. How can you determine whether your patient's symptoms result from stress or from hypovolemic shock?

If you can answer yes to two or more of the following questions, suspect hypovolemic shock and notify the doctor immediately.
• Is the patient's skin cool, clammy, and pale?
• Is he restless, anxious, or confused?
• Is his pulse rapid and thready?
• Is his pulse pressure narrowing?
• Is his urine output low (less than 30 ml/hour)?
• Are his sensory perceptions diminished?

Nursing interventions. Your patient will need emergency intervention to improve ventilation and replace lost fluids. In addition to carefully assessing and monitoring his vital signs, take these other nursing measures during treatment:
• Check for a patent airway and adequate circulation. If pulse and blood pressure are absent, begin CPR.
• Place the patient in a supine position. If he's hemorrhaging severely, elevate his legs 20° to 30°.
• Record blood pressure, pulse rate, peripheral pulses, and respiratory rate and other vital signs every 15 minutes. If systolic blood pressure drops below 80 mm Hg, notify the doctor immediately.
• Monitor the EKG continuously.
• As ordered, start I.V.s with normal saline or lactated Ringer's solution, using a large-bore catheter for easier administration of later blood transfusions. (*Caution:* If your patient in shock has suffered abdominal trauma, in addition to chest trauma, don't start I.V.s in the legs, since infused fluid may escape through the ruptured vessel into the abdomen.)
• If certified, draw blood for arterial blood gas measurements. Administer oxygen by face mask or airway to ensure adequate tissue oxygenation. Adjust the oxygen flow rate according to ABG values.
• Administer oxygen by face mask or airway to ensure adequate tissue oxygenation.
• The doctor may want to measure the patient's hourly urinary output with a Foley catheter. If output remains below 30 ml/hour, notify the doctor.
• Assess the patient's skin color and temperature frequently. Cold, clammy skin may indicate progressive shock.
• Watch for signs of impending coagulopathy (for example, bruising, petechiae, or bleeding or oozing from the gums or venipuncture site).
• Explain all procedures and provide emotional support to the patient and his family.

CHEST CONTUSION

SETTING THE SCENE

Late one summer evening, paramedics wheel Chris Paone into the emergency department (ED). According to witnesses, Chris, a tall, slight, 19-year-old, was driving north on the expressway when he swerved to avoid hitting a dog.

The policeman accompanying him provides the details: Chris apparently lost control of his car and slammed into a guard rail. The sudden stop threw him against the steering wheel so violently that the wheel cracked in two. When the police arrived at the scene, they found Chris (who wasn't wearing a seat belt) unconscious and bleeding from multiple lacerations on his head and face.

Based on this and other information from the police report, the ED nurses immediately suspect chest contusion and begin lifesaving measures. Are the nurses' suspicions and actions well-founded? To answer the question, consider these facts:

As the term implies, chest contusion results from a forceful blow that compresses the thoracic cavity. In Chris' case, the blow was produced by the steering wheel. In most cases, such a blow injures the patient's heart (as in myocardial contusion) or the lungs (as in pulmonary contusion), or both.

The injury's severity depends on chest wall flexibility and the amount of thoracic wall padding. An obese patient, for example, is less likely to sustain severe chest contusion than a thinner patient like Chris. But regardless of the severity, myocardial and pulmonary contusions pose special problems. Unless they're recognized and treated quickly, these injuries can lead to fatal complications. And despite their serious nature, chest contusions may remain asymptomatic for days or even weeks.

Consequently, when caring for a patient with a chest contusion, suspect intrathoracic injuries. These hidden injuries may be more serious than visible ones.

Nearly 40% of chest trauma victims don't survive. But on the next few pages, we'll explain how to keep a chest contusion patient like Chris on the surviving side of that statistic.

PULMONARY CONTUSION: THE COMPRESSION–DECOMPRESSION INJURY

When assessing any patient with blunt chest trauma, consider the possibility of pulmonary contusion: 30% to 75% of patients with blunt chest trauma have this condition. In some cases, the injury is mild and may be overshadowed by other injuries such as flail chest, pneumothorax, or hemothorax.

However, pulmonary contusion kills up to 40% of its victims. To survive this injury, the patient needs aggressive treatment. To understand the urgency, consider how this chest trauma affects respiratory function.

Pulmonary contusion is caused by a high-pressure injury that compresses the lung by diminishing thorax size. (Steering wheel accidents are a frequent cause of such an injury.) As the compressing force is removed, decompression occurs, creating a momentary negative intrathoracic pressure. This pressure change further injures the lung areas initially damaged during compression. Blood leaks into the alveoli, causing hemorrhage and pulmonary edema.

As the edema worsens and cellular debris accumulates, gas exchange suffers and interstitial pressure rises. Eventually, atelectasis occurs, pulmonary vascular resistance rises, and pulmonary arterial pressure increases. In addition, because of impaired gas exchange, pulmonary blood flow decreases. Ultimately, the patient develops systemic hypoxia and hypercapnia. If the contused area's large enough, the patient may die from hypoxia, even with early and aggressive treatment.

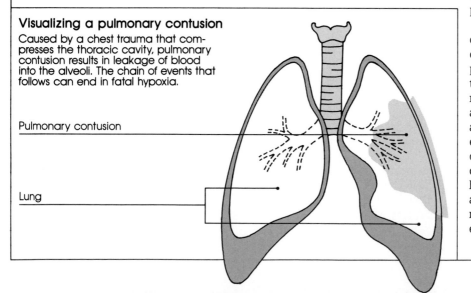

Visualizing a pulmonary contusion

Caused by a chest trauma that compresses the thoracic cavity, pulmonary contusion results in leakage of blood into the alveoli. The chain of events that follows can end in fatal hypoxia.

Pulmonary contusion

Lung

ASSESSING THE INJURY

Signs and symptoms of pulmonary contusion are usually well-defined. You can classify most pulmonary contusions as mild, moderate, or severe, according to physical findings. For a convenient comparison of the signs and symptoms of pulmonary contusion types, study the chart below:

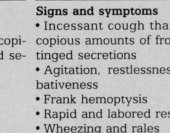

MILD PULMONARY CONTUSION
Signs and symptoms • Chest pain • Loose cough that produces copious and possibly blood-tinged secretions. • Tachypnea • Tachycardia • Loose rales

MODERATE PULMONARY CONTUSION
Signs and symptoms • Incessant cough that doesn't clear secretions

• Frank bleeding in the tracheobronchial tree
• Labored respirations
• Restlessness
• Apprehension
• Progressive respiratory insufficiency with dyspnea, tachypnea, and cyanosis

SEVERE PULMONARY CONTUSION
Signs and symptoms • Incessant cough that produces copious amounts of frothy, blood-tinged secretions • Agitation, restlessness, or combativeness • Frank hemoptysis • Rapid and labored respirations • Wheezing and rales • Bronchial breath sounds • Tachycardia • Cyanosis

CONFIRMING THE DIAGNOSIS

To confirm physical findings in a patient with suspected pulmonary contusion, the doctor will probably order chest X-rays. If pulmonary contusion has occurred, X-rays will show one of two basic patterns.

The most frequent pattern shows patchy, ill-defined areas of increased parenchymal density, reflecting intraalveolar hemorrhage. In a mild contusion, this pattern may appear only in a few local areas. In moderate-to-severe contusion, the pattern may cover extensive areas of one or both lungs.

A severely contused lung will also appear larger than the unaffected lung from edema. The affected lung's increased weight pushes the diaphragm downward,

possibly causing gastrointestinal distention. A less common pattern shows linear and irregular bronchial infiltrates.

When assessing a patient for pulmonary contusion, keep in mind that, despite the injury's severity, abnormalities may not appear on chest X-rays for 24 to 48 hours after the accident. Consequently, subsequent X-rays may be necessary. You may also find it difficult to recognize signs and symptoms of hypoxia, especially in patients with multiple injuries. To accurately evaluate your patient's gas exchange, obtain arterial blood gas measurements.

MANAGING THE PATIENT

The key to managing pulmonary contusion is providing good tracheobronchial care, including intratracheal suctioning and chest physiotherapy, as ordered. Additional measures depend on the severity of the patient's injury and his particular needs.

Mild pulmonary contusion. In most cases, the doctor begins treatment by ordering oxygen (by mask or nasal cannula) for 24 to 36 hours, endotracheal suctioning, and narcotics to relieve the pain. For patients with severe pain, he may perform an intercostal nerve block.

If secretions remain despite suctioning, he may order bronchoscopy. If bronchospasm occurs, ultrasonic nebulization by mist, with a bronchodilator such as isoetharine hydrochloride 1% or metaproterenol sulfate, is usually necessary. A patient with gastrointestinal distention may need a nasogastric tube connected to low suction.

Since a damaged lung is susceptible to infection, the doctor may order broad-spectrum antibiotics. Obtain sputum cultures as ordered, and administer antibiotics accordingly. Restrict fluids, according to doctor's orders, to avoid fluid overload.

Most patients with mild pulmonary contusion recover within 72 to 96 hours after receiving treatment. However, observe the patient carefully throughout treatment for complications such as pulmonary embolism or pneumonia.

Moderate pulmonary contusion. A patient with this injury usually requires mechanical ventilation through an endotracheal tube to remove secretions and reduce the work of breathing. Repositioning the patient regularly will also help loosen and remove se-

CONTINUED ON PAGE 112

CHEST CONTUSION CONTINUED

MANAGING THE PATIENT
CONTINUED

cretions. Blood transfusions with whole blood or packed cells may also be required to achieve adequate hemoglobin levels, since hemoglobin enhances oxygen transport to body tissues.

To prevent fluid overload, the doctor will probably restrict the patient's fluid intake to approximately 50 ml/hour. To decrease excess fluid, he may also order diuretics and serum albumin. Large doses of steroids may be required, too. Studies show that these drugs reduce the contusion's size.

A patient with moderate pulmonary contusion usually recovers within 10 to 14 days, at which time he can be weaned from the ventilator. If the contusion doesn't resolve after that time, suspect complications such as pneumonia or pulmonary embolism. Despite early intervention, about 15% of patients with moderate pulmonary contusion die.

Severe pulmonary contusion.
Early signs of respiratory failure may appear in a patient with this injury. A common treatment is ventilating the patient with high-flow oxygen, then waiting and treating any complications that may arise.

But despite early and aggressive treatment (similar to that for moderate pulmonary contusion), a patient with severe pulmonary contusion deteriorates rapidly. Death from hypoxia usually occurs within 72 to 96 hours after the injury.

MYOCARDIAL CONTUSION: THE UNDERDIAGNOSED INJURY

Because myocardial contusion may be well-tolerated and occur without any external signs of injury, it's commonly overlooked in patients with multiple trauma.

After a contusion, hemorrhage occurs within the myocardium. In a large contusion, the heart's contractility, cardiac output, and blood pressure diminish. Perfusion abnormalities also occur, resulting in hypoxia. As the heart tries to compensate for excessive ventricular blood volume, tachycardia develops. Without prompt treatment, the patient will undergo cardiogenic shock.

Assessment. Begin by taking a thorough history. Myocardial contusion's likely in any patient who sustains chest trauma from a steering wheel injury, blows from a fist or club, a high-altitude fall, or impact with cycle handlebars.

Although physical findings for myocardial contusion may be scarce, two signs suggest this injury in any patient with blunt chest trauma: tachycardia and bruises over the sternum.

The patient may also complain of precordial pain that mimics the pain of myocardial infarction. However, contusion pain isn't relived by coronary vasodilators.

Management. The goal of management is to restore and maintain normal cardiac function. The doctor will probably order a mild analgesic to relieve chest pain and place the patient on bed rest with restricted activity for 2 to 4 weeks. During this period, take the following nursing actions:
• Monitor the patient's fluid intake.
• Check central venous pressure or pulmonary capillary wedge pressure.
• Monitor his EKG and cardiac output.

FRACTURES

RIB FRACTURES: SIMPLE TO COMPLEX

Rib fracture, the most common chest injury, can seriously threaten a patient's respiratory status. The more ribs involved and the greater the rib displacement, the more critical the patient's condition. A rib may be displaced either inward, toward the lungs; or outward, away from them.

On the following pages you'll learn:
• how to recognize the various rib fracture types
• which complications to anticipate
• which nursing measures to take for each fracture type.

Simple fractures. In most cases, rib fracture results from an injury (such as a fall), a blow to the chest, or—the most common cause—the impact of being thrown against a car's steering wheel. In a simple fracture, the injury's force distributes over a wide area of the chest wall. The affected rib buckles outward and breaks—usually in midshaft position—without puncturing the lung.

From fall to fracture. Robert Gannon, a 27-year-old contractor, is admitted to the hospital with a torn meniscus after falling from a ladder. Following a whirlpool session, Mr. Gannon slips while getting out of the bath, falling on his left side. He assures the physical therapist he feels fine.

But less than 2 hours later, he complains of severe pain in his left side—a pain that worsens when he breathes deeply or tries to reposition himself in bed. Since the therapist informed you of Mr. Gannon's fall, you immediately suspect a fractured rib.

A physical assessment confirms your suspicion: While palpating, you note extreme tenderness in Mr. Gannon's left side at his fifth rib; you also feel bone crepitus.

You notify Mr. Gannon's doctor, who orders an analgesic for pain relief. (For a patient with excruciating pain, the doctor may order an I.M. narcotic, such as codeine, or perform an intercostal nerve block.)

The doctor also orders chest X-rays. Since anterior and lateral rib fractures aren't always visible on a routine chest X-ray, he may request views of the left and right anterior oblique angles or rib films in addition to the standard views. For any patient with suspected rib fracture, the doctor will probably order inspiratory and expiratory posteroanterior chest X-rays to rule out pneumothorax and other complications. *Note:* Any patient whose physical examination suggests a rib fracture should receive treatment for a fracture regardless of chest X-ray findings.

For an otherwise healthy patient like Mr. Gannon, the doctor may also order adhesive chest strapping. In such a patient, the strapping probably won't impede coughing and deep-breathing exercises that help prevent the mucous accumulation that can lead to pneumonia.

Simple fractures, special situations. A patient who's elderly or who has preexisting lung disease or a low pain threshold stands a greater chance of developing respiratory complications in association with a fractured rib.

To understand why, consider the asthmatic patient who fractures a rib. Because deep breathing aggravates his severe pain, he resorts to shallow breathing in an attempt to minimize chest wall expansion. As a result, fewer alveoli are perfused. If diminished perfusion continues, alveoli collapse, secretions accumulate, and atelectasis sets in—exacerbating the asthma.

To make matters worse, the patient also coughs less to avoid aggravating the pain. This impairs secretion removal and worsens his asthma. Unless interrupted, these developments can trigger a vicious cycle of deterioration, leading to pneumonia or even respiratory failure.

These special patients usually need more aggressive care. In most cases, the doctor will order a narcotic such as codeine, administered in low doses to control pain without depressing respirations. He'll probably also perform an intercostal nerve block.

Nursing measures. To ensure that the patient with a rib fracture has adequate lung perfusion and minimal secretions, the doctor will probably instruct you to perform endotracheal suctioning and administer ultrasonic nebulization by mist.

While providing tracheobronchial care for a patient with a fractured rib, culture his secretions frequently for laboratory evaluation. If necessary, administer antibiotics as ordered.

Once the patient's pain abates—which usually takes 5 to 7 days—the doctor will probably begin oral analgesic therapy. The rib fracture should heal completely within 6 weeks.

STERNUM FRACTURES

Sternum fractures, caused by severe trauma to the front of the chest, are usually accompanied by various cardiac and intrathoracic injuries—many of them life-threatening. Your goals in caring for a patient with a fractured sternum are usually two-fold: First, manage the associated injury, since this poses the greatest threat; then, treat the sternum fracture. Associated injuries include flail chest, pulmonary and myocardial contusion, hemothorax and pneumothorax, and cardiac and spinal injuries.

Assessment. The patient with a displaced sternum fracture usually complains of a sharp, stabbing pain. His chest may be tender, swollen, and discolored over the fracture site; you may also feel crepitus. To confirm the diagnosis, the doctor will probably order a lateral or oblique chest X-ray.

Note: If the sternum fracture's not displaced, the patient may be asymptomatic and the fracture may go undetected.

Management. Most sternum fractures occur near the manubrium, the sternum's fixed, unyielding, uppermost portion. Consequently, an impact injury to the lower two thirds of the sternum usually displaces the sternum forward, away from the manubrium.

Once the associated injuries have been controlled, the sternum fracture will be treated. Therapy varies according to the fracture's severity. For example, a patient with a sternum fracture that's not displaced may require only analgesics for pain relief. However, if his pain is severe, the doctor may perform an intercostal nerve block.

A patient with a severe sternum fracture will probably require operative stabilization (also called surgical fixation).

FRACTURES CONTINUED

MULTIPLE FRACTURES AND FLAIL CHEST

Respiratory complications can occur in a patient with even a single fractured rib. But for a patient with multiple rib fractures, acute respiratory distress is almost a certainty. The reason: The patient may develop flail chest, which results from fractured ribs or a fractured sternum, or both. Each involved rib breaks in at least two places. The resulting segmentation allows the fractured region to free itself from the normally rigid chest wall, and to flail in response to intrathoracic pressure rather than to the pull of respiratory muscles. The result is paradoxical chest wall movement.

Normally, the chest wall expands during inspiration, producing a negative pressure inside the chest that allows air to be sucked in. During normal expiration, the chest wall retracts, creating a positive intrathoracic pressure that forces air out.

In flail chest, the unstable, or flail, part is also sucked in during inspiration, then forced outward during expiration. Consequently, the lung tissue underlying the flail part can't expand and fill with air on inspiration—a situation ripe for atelectasis.

Check carefully for signs of posterior flail chest. Because the patient's usually supine during an examination, you may overlook this injury.

Paradoxical chest movement's most severe with anterior fractures, particularly transverse sternal fractures and those that separate the ribs from the sternum. In lateral and posterior flail chest, paradoxical movement's less marked.

Complications. Flail chest poses two immediate risks. A fractured rib could puncture a lung, causing pneumothorax, hemothorax, or tension pneumothorax. Flail chest can also cause hypoxia, which can lead to respiratory failure if untreated.

MANAGING FLAIL CHEST

If you suspect your patient has flail chest, stabilize the segment by positioning him on his affected side, or place pillows or sandbags over the injury. Once the doctor has confirmed flail chest, he'll probably order morphine to reduce the patient's pain, then perform an intercostal nerve block. In most cases, he'll also perform endotracheal intubation and order mechanical ventilation.

If the patient's not on a ventilator, the doctor will probably order nasotracheal suctioning and continued oxygen administration to maintain adequate PaO$_2$ levels. To ensure good pulmonary care, take the following measures:
• Keep the patient in an upright position to help improve lung expansion. At least every 2 hours, change his position by logrolling him to provide stability and comfort. Try to turn him to his unaffected side when possible to improve alveolar perfusion. If he has posterior rib fractures, don't position him on his back.
• If possible, have the patient cough and deep breathe at least every 2 hours. To encourage him to perform these exercises more frequently, give him a pillow to splint tender sites.
• If he's intubated, suction him vigorously. (But remember to hyperoxygenate him first.)
Balancing fluids. Managing fluid in the flail chest patient is essential. Any lost blood must be replaced with whole or packed red blood cells. And because a contused lung handles water poorly (since body fluid shifts from intravascular to extravascular spaces around damaged tissue), the patient may need plasma or serum albumin to maintain fluid volume. These colloidal fluids keep fluid in the pulmonary capillaries, helping to maintain adequate circulation.

Paradoxical chest movement

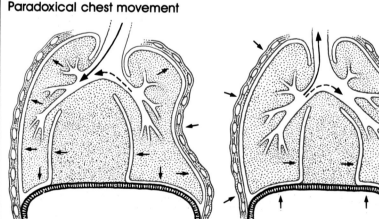
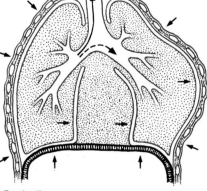

Inspiration
The chest wall normally expands during inspiration, drawing air into the lungs. But in flail chest, the flail section retracts as the patient inspires, as shown in the illustration above. Atelectasis sets in as lung tissue beneath the injury can't expand.

Expiration
As the illustration above shows, the flail area moves in a direction opposite to the rest of the chest wall, bulging out during expiration. Consequently, the patient can't expel air effectively.

PNEUMOTHORAX

During the initial treatment stage, avoid administering crystalloid I.V. fluids such as normal saline solution or dextrose 5% in water. These fluids leak out of pulmonary capillaries surrounding damaged tissue and worsen preexisting pulmonary edema.

The doctor will probably ask you to monitor your patient's hematocrit to assess his fluid status and monitor his intake and output to assess fluid balance.

Throughout your care, observe the patient often for cyanosis, respiratory distress, and changes in mental status. Evaluate bilateral breath sounds routinely for presence, intensity, and adventitious sounds. Also review his ABG values frequently to assess his ventilation.

SURGICAL FIXATION
Some patients with rib and sternum fractures—especially multiple fractures that cause paradoxical chest movement—may need surgical intervention to facilitate adequate ventilation and prevent further respiratory deterioration. This procedure, which may be external or internal, may reduce or eliminate the patient's need for endotracheal intubation and mechanical ventilation.
External fixation. The doctor stabilizes the patient's fracture by inserting pins through the overlying skin directly into the fractured rib. He then connects the pins to an external framework that he tightens to align and immobilize the fracture.
Internal fixation. Through an incision, the doctor inserts metal pins or wires that bind the fractured ribs together. This method enables the doctor to correct associated intrathoracic injuries and reconstruct damaged portions of the chest wall.

PNEUMOTHORAX: PLEURAL CAVITY AIR TRAP
Simply speaking, pneumothorax is a collection of air or gas in the normally airtight pleural cavity. Left untreated, this respiratory emergency leads to lung compression and collapse, in turn reducing tidal volume, impairing gas exchange, and threatening your patient's life. Pneumothorax is classified according to cause: spontaneous, traumatic, or tension.
Spontaneous pneumothorax. This crisis occurs when air enters the pleural cavity through an opening in the lung surface. Also known as closed pneumothorax because the chest wall remains closed, spontaneous pneumothorax may be *primary* or *secondary.*

Primary spontaneous pneumothorax arises unexpectedly in an otherwise healthy adult between ages 20 and 40. In most cases, it results from an undetected alveolar bleb (small vesicle) or bulla (large vesicle) on the lung. Excessive stress, for example, from coughing or exercising, may cause the bleb to rupture, creating an opening that allows air to seep from the lungs into the pleural cavity.

Although blebs most commonly develop in the lung apices, autopsies frequently reveal them in areas of undetected paraseptal emphysema bordering the pleura.

Secondary spontaneous pneumothorax, which also develops unexpectedly, usually results from a disorder that hyperinflates the lungs, such as asthma or emphysema. However, in some cases, it's caused by an anatomic deformity, such as pulmonary fibrosis, or by a tubercular or malignant lesion that has eroded into the pleural space.
Sizing a spontaneous pneumothorax. A spontaneous pneumothorax may be small, moderate,
CONTINUED ON PAGE 116

Pneumothorax types

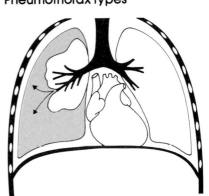

Spontaneous pneumothorax
The chest wall remains intact in this injury. Air (shown in blue in the illustration above) enters the normally airtight pleural cavity through the lung's surface.

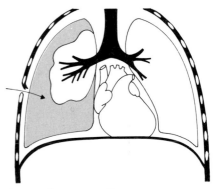

Traumatic pneumothorax
This disorder results from entry of air into the pleural space through a chest wall opening.

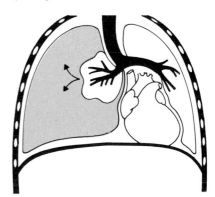

Tension pneumothorax
When an increasing amount of air becomes trapped in the pleural space, a tension pneumothorax may develop. As air and tension increase, the lung and mediastinum are compressed and shifted toward the unaffected side.

PNEUMOTHORAX CONTINUED

PNEUMOTHORAX: PLEURAL CAVITY AIR TRAP
CONTINUED

or large, depending on the percentage of the pleural cavity filled with air. In most cases, only patients with moderate or large pneumothoraces experience signs and symptoms.
• Small spontaneous pneumothorax: 15% or less
• Moderate spontaneous pneumothorax: 15% to 60%
• Large spontaneous pneumothorax: 60% or more

Traumatic pneumothorax. This disorder follows an external chest wall injury, which creates a chest wall opening that permits direct communication between the atmosphere and the pleural cavity. Traumatic pneumothorax may result from a penetrating chest wound inflicted by a knife or gunshot, or from lung puncture caused by a blow that fractures a rib and pushes it inward. It may also be caused by a medical procedure such as central venous pressure line insertion, thoracic surgery, thoracentesis, or mechanical ventilation with PEEP.

Tension pneumothorax. A life-threatening complication of spontaneous or traumatic pneumothorax, tension pneumothorax occurs when air enters the pleural cavity and can't escape. With each inspiration, more air becomes trapped, increasing intrathoracic pressure. This growing pressure can shift mediastinal structures to the unaffected side, compressing the opposite lung and leading to acute respiratory distress.

In time, mediastinal shift causes the great vessels to form a sharp obstructive angle, which reduces venous return, cardiac output, and blood pressure. Undetected, tension pneumothorax can cause death from hypoxia and respiratory acidosis.

RECOGNIZING SIGNS AND SYMPTOMS

A patient with a small pneumothorax may not experience any signs or symptoms. A patient with a tension pneumothorax or a mild-to-moderate spontaneous or traumatic pneumothorax may have the following signs and symptoms:
• sudden, sharp pain on the affected side that increases with chest movement, coughing, and breathing and may radiate to the shoulder
• asymmetric chest wall movement
• shortness of breath
• anxiety
• subcutaneous emphysema in the neck and upper chest
• cyanosis
• rapid pulse and respiratory rate
• sucking sound near the wound (in open pneumothorax)
• neck vein distention (in large pneumothorax).

History. A patient's chest pain and shortness of breath may cause you to confuse pneumothorax with myocardial ischemia, a dissecting aortic aneurysm, or pulmonary embolism. To help rule out these disorders, take a thorough history.

Physical examination. While examining your patient, check for decreased or absent chest movement and breath sounds on the affected side. Auscultate for decreased or absent breath sounds over the collapsed lung. However, keep in mind that pain and splinting will affect these sounds.

Percuss for hyperresonance and decreased tactile fremitus on the affected side. Palpate for tracheal deviation to the unaffected side and crackling under the skin—which indicates subcutaneous emphysema—and for decreased vocal fremitus on the affected side.

Diagnostic tests. The doctor will probably order the following tests to confirm pneumothorax:
• *Chest X-ray.* This test will probably reveal a lowered diaphragm, air in the pleural cavity, chest wall expansion, and partial or total lung collapse on the affected side.
• *Arterial blood gases (ABGs).* These values usually show PaO_2 less than 80 mm Hg, $PaCO_2$ less than 35 mm Hg, and pH greater than 7.45, indicating hypoxemia and respiratory alkalosis.

ANTICIPATING COMPLICATIONS

Before your patient's pneumothorax resolves, he may develop complications such as hemothorax, pleural effusion, and empyema.

To help prevent potentially fatal complications, stay alert for the following danger signs:
• increased respiratory rate, dyspnea, unusual chest movement, and abnormal breath sounds, which may indicate a new air leak in the lungs or incomplete air evacuation from the pleural cavity
• increased pulse, respiratory rate, and temperature; or behavioral changes, which may be an early sign of a developing complication
• changes in drainage color or quantity. Sanguineous drainage indicates hemothorax; straw-colored drainage signifies pleural effusion; purulent drainage indicates empyema.

If your patient develops any of these complications, reassure him frequently, since anxiety will exacerbate his chest pain and any breathing difficulty.

INTERVENTION: THREE GOALS

While caring for the pneumothorax patient, keep the following goals in mind: relieve acute distress, monitor signs and symptoms, and prevent complications. Follow the guidelines below:

• Provide emotional support and make the patient as comfortable as possible (he'll usually prefer a sitting position). Explain what pneumothorax is, and let him know which treatments to expect.

• Monitor his vital signs at least once an hour for indications of shock, increasing respiratory distress, or mediastinal shift. Auscultate breath sounds over both lungs. Remember—falling blood pressure and rising pulse and respiratory rates may indicate tension pneumothorax.

• Keep a thoracostomy tray at the patient's bedside. The doctor may perform this procedure to relieve chest pressure.

• Encourage the patient to deep breathe to reexpand the lung.

• As ordered, administer medications to control pain and promote coughing and deep breathing. Drugs such as acetaminophen 300 mg with codeine (Tylenol with Codeine No. 3), oxycodone hydrochloride (Percocet**), and propoxyphene napsylate (Darvocet-N*) don't depress respiratory function.

• If the pneumothorax is small, monitor the patient's vital signs, respiratory status, and general condition. Note signs of increasing respiratory distress that could indicate an increasing pneumothorax.

• If the pneumothorax is moderate or large, or if the patient's symptomatic, prepare to assist with chest-tube insertion. Urge the patient to control coughing and gasping during the procedure.

Chest-tube nursing measures. If your patient has a chest tube, take these steps:

• Watch for continuing air leakage (bubbling), a sign that the lung defect remains open. Check for increasing subcutaneous emphysema. Palpate around the patient's neck or at the chest-tube insertion site to check for crepitus. If he's on a ventilator, check for difficulty breathing in time with the ventilator, as well as pressure changes on ventilator gauges.

• Change dressings around the chest-tube insertion site as needed. Take care not to reposition or displace the tube.

• Provide emotional support to the patient and his family.

• Monitor vital signs frequently. For the first 24 hours, check breath sounds every hour to assess the patient's respiratory status. Observe the insertion site for leakage and note the amount and color of drainage.

• Arrange for follow-up chest X-rays, as needed, to assess lung reexpansion.

*Not available in Canada

**Not available in the United States

INSERTING AND REMOVING A CHEST TUBE

If your pneumothorax patient's experiencing any respiratory problems, regardless of pneumothorax size, the doctor will insert a chest tube to reexpand the lung.

Like any drain, a chest tube removes unwanted materials—in this case, air or liquid in the pleural cavity. It also helps prevent air or liquid from returning.

Before insertion, administer a sedative, as ordered. Tell the patient what's going to be done and why. After the tube's inserted and the drainage system is hooked up, encourage the patient to deep breathe and exhale fully to help drain the pleural space and reexpand the lung. Make sure a chest X-ray has been ordered to check the tube's position and effectiveness.

Assess the patient regularly, paying particular attention to his respiratory status.

Removal. Expect the doctor to remove the chest tube when a chest X-ray reveals full lung expansion or as little as 5% air remaining in the pleural cavity. This usually occurs within 3 days of chest-tube insertion.

About 24 hours before removing the tube, the doctor may ask you to clamp it to assess the patient's tolerance. When the tube's clamped, closely monitor the patient for signs and symptoms of respiratory distress, which may indicate that some air remains in the pleural cavity. Arrange for a chest X-ray approximately 2 hours after clamping to assess pleural cavity integrity.

If the patient develops respiratory distress, or if the chest X-ray reveals recurrent pneumothorax, immediately unclamp the tube, reestablish suction, and notify the doctor.

If the patient tolerates clamping, the doctor will remove the chest tube. Administer an analgesic as ordered, and place the patient in semi-Fowler's position or on his unaffected side, according to the doctor's instructions.

Observation. For the first few hours after chest-tube removal, closely monitor your patient's vital signs and observe respiratory quality and depth. Call the doctor if you detect any abnormalities.

PNEUMOTHORAX CONTINUED

THORACIC DRAINAGE SYSTEMS: YOUR RESPONSIBILITIES

No matter which thoracic drainage system the doctor orders for your patient, the basic principles are the same: by providing gravity, and in some cases suction, the system restores negative intrapleural pressure and removes any air or blood trapped in the pleural cavity.

A drainage system may consist of a one-bottle underwater seal, a two-bottle (Emerson) setup, a three-bottle (Pleur-evac or Thora-Drain III) setup, or a four-bottle (Argyle) setup.

Nursing care. When caring for a patient with a chest tube connected to a drainage system, you're responsible for maintaining a closed sterile system to prevent passage of air or pathogens into the pleural cavity. After emptying the drainage system or changing the bottles, check for an underwater seal to ensure that no additional air will enter the pleural cavity.

To promote drainage and prevent additional pressure buildup, keep the tubing patent. To do this, check for kinks in the tubing and make sure the suction level is maintained as ordered. If the suction level's too low, accumulated air can't be completely removed from the pleural cavity. Usually 20 to 30 cm of thoracic suction restores negative pressure.

Goals. Consider thoracic drainage effective if the patient breathes more easily, his color returns, his chest pain subsides, and his apprehension diminishes.

Thora-Drain III
A disposable underwater-seal chest drainage system, such as the Thora-Drain III shown below, saves time and eliminates the risk of bottle breakage. The basic three-bottle setup is enclosed in one unit.

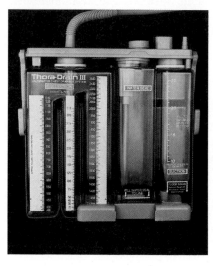

The Heimlich flutter valve
As shown in the illustration below, the Heimlich flutter valve allows air and drainage to escape from the pleural cavity while preventing air reentry. The valve is attached as shown after the chest tube's clamped and disconnected from the drainage system. A sterile dressing or a sterile glove with a puncture for accumulated air attaches to the end of the valve to collect drainage.

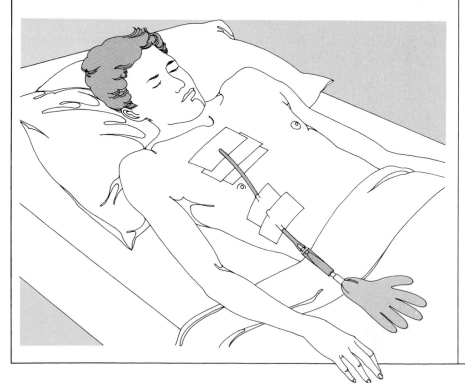

USING A FLUTTER VALVE
A patient who has a small, slowly resolving pneumothorax or who requires transfer to another floor may require a flutter valve. The doctor may also insert a flutter valve as a temporary measure before chest-tube insertion until he connects the chest tube to a drainage system. The Heimlich flutter valve, for example, allows trapped air and drainage to escape from the pleural cavity during expiration without allowing additional air to enter during inspiration.

To attach a flutter valve, the doctor clamps the chest tube and disconnects it from the drainage system, then positions and secures the valve in the direction of the flow. To collect drainage, he'll place a sterile glove or dressing on the end of the valve.

THE McSWAIN DART SYSTEM: THE CHEST TUBE ALTERNATIVE

The McSwain Dart System is replacing the chest tube for many pneumothorax patients—particularly those with spontaneous nontension pneumothorax. It consists of a stainless steel stylet attached to a French catheter, polyvinylchloride drainage tubing, and an injection-molded valve (see photo below).

Insertion. The dart's usually inserted at the second intercostal space at the midclavicular line, or at the third or fourth intercostal space at the anterior axillary line, on the affected side. If the pneumothorax isn't life-threatening, the doctor may anesthetize the insertion site first.

The doctor makes a small incision and advances the dart (with its wings closed) through the skin into the chest cavity. When he feels a pop, he'll know he's reached the pleural cavity and will advance the dart ¼″ (0.5 cm). At this point, he'll withdraw the stylet ⅜″ (1 cm) and advance the dart another ⅝″ (1.5 cm). Next he removes the stylet.

After the dart's connected to the tubing attached to the inline one-way valve, the doctor will secure the device by holding the dart's flared fitting while advancing the housing to extend the wings. When the dart's secured, urge your patient to cough. As he does so, make sure air escapes through the one-way valve. Apply low suction to the valve, if ordered. To evacuate the pleural cavity as thoroughly as possible, the doctor will retract the device against the chest wall, then tape or sew it in place to prevent accidental dislodgement.

Postinsertion care. After the system's in place, keep the tubing patent and free of kinks. Check your patient's vital signs frequently and report any abnormal changes to the doctor.

The McSwain Dart System

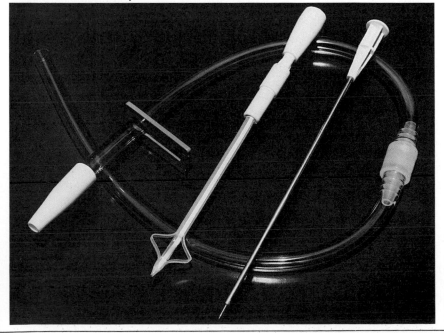

DETECTING A RECURRENCE: PATIENT-TEACHING TIPS

If your patient has a spontaneous pneumothorax, he has a 60% chance of experiencing a recurrence on the same or opposite side. Pneumothorax may recur a few days after the initial pneumothorax—or up to 20 years later. However, it usually recurs within 2 to 3 years.

To prepare your patient for a recurrence, explain the risk and answer any questions he and his family may have. Emphasize the importance of detecting telltale signs and symptoms early and seeking medical attention immediately. Instruct him to watch for these indications:
• sharp, stabbing chest pain
• shortness of breath
• anxiety or restlessness
• increased pulse and respiration rate.

PNEUMOTHORAX RECURRENCE: TREATMENT OPTIONS

Has your patient's pneumothorax persisted for more than 7 days despite chest tube insertion and drainage? Or, has he developed a new pneumothorax after discharge? The doctor may perform a thoracotomy to suture or staple the leak, to make pleural abrasions, or to resect the defective lung area.

Recurring spontaneous pneumothorax can also be treated with pleurodesis. In this procedure, an irritating substance such as tetracycline, talc, or kaolin is instilled between the visceral and parietal pleurae during a thoracostomy. The pleural adhesions that result help prevent pneumothorax recurrence.

HEMOTHORAX

HEMOTHORAX BASICS

One evening when you're on duty in the E.D., ambulance attendants wheel in Burton Collier, age 27. The victim of a barroom stabbing, Mr. Collier's bleeding heavily from a chest wound.

After making sure his airway's open and he's breathing adequately, you quickly cover the wound with a gauze bandage in case the wound has caused a pneumothorax.

During your assessment, Mr. Collier complains of chest pain, hemoptysis, tachypnea, and dyspnea. Because you immediately suspect hemothorax resulting from the stab wound, you call the doctor. (*Note:* Hemothorax can also result from blunt chest trauma.)

Based on your physical findings, patient history, blood studies, and a chest X-ray, the doctor confirms that Mr. Collier has a hemothorax.

Defining hemothorax. Hemothorax develops when blood leaks into the pleural cavity from a damaged lung, the heart, the great vessels and their branches,

an intercostal artery or vein, a mediastinal vein, or the vessels of the diaphragm or chest wall. When a large volume of blood accumulates in the pleural cavity, circulating fluid volume decreases, causing hypovolemia.

About 25% of patients with blunt or penetrating chest trauma have hemothorax.

The patient also experiences diminished cardiac output, hypotension, and eventually metabolic acidosis. As his circulatory system quickly becomes depleted from impaired gas exchange and circulatory functions, he becomes a candidate for hypovolemic shock. Soon, the accumulating blood compresses the involved lung, reducing ventilation and causing hypoxia.

Another hemothorax characteristic is mediastinal shift. A large blood buildup in the pleural cavity causes the mediastinum to shift toward the uninvolved lung.

Under normal conditions, the uninvolved lung attempts to compensate for the damaged one. But mediastinal shift interferes with existing lung function and aggravates ventilatory problems. Left untreated, the combination of hypovolemia and hypoxia can kill. In many cases, pneumothorax accompanies hemothorax, compounding the risk.

Risk factors. About one of every four patients with blunt or penetrating chest trauma has hemothorax. A hemothorax may also occur from thoracic surgery, pulmonary infarction, neoplasm, dissecting thoracic aneurysm, or anticoagulant therapy.

HOW HEMOTHORAX SIZE AFFECTS SIGNS AND SYMPTOMS

A common method of classifying hemothorax is by size—small, moderate, or massive. Hemothorax size determines which signs and symptoms your patient will develop and how much blood is lost. Consequently, you can usually estimate the seriousness of your patient's injury if you know how large the hemothorax is. Use the chart below to compare signs and symptoms and diagnostic findings for each hemothorax size.

SMALL HEMOTHORAX

Approximate blood loss
Less than 400 ml

Signs and symptoms
Usually none

Diagnostic findings
• With less than 250 ml of accumulated fluid, no recognizable chest X-ray changes. With 250 to 400 ml of fluid, chest X-ray shows blunting of costophrenic angle.

MODERATE HEMOTHORAX

Approximate blood loss
500 to 2,000 ml

Signs and symptoms
• Indications of internal hemorrhage (such as pallor, restlessness, anxiety, tachycardia, and decreased blood pressure)
• Dyspnea
• Chest tightening
• Asymmetrical chest movement
• Ecchymosis over the affected lung
• Bloody sputum

Visualizing a hemothorax

Trauma to the chest wall, lung tissue, or mediastinum can cause a hemothorax—leakage of blood into the pleural space (as shown on the left in the illustration below).

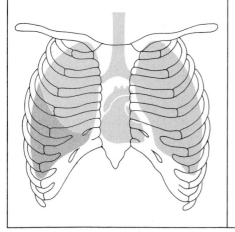

Diagnostic findings
• Dullness over the affected side heard during percussion
• Decreased or absent breath sounds over the affected side heard during auscultation; exaggerated bronchovesicular breath sounds above fluid level (less common)
• Decreased tactile fremitus over the affected side noted during palpation
• Decreased hemoglobin (less common)
• Blood or serosanguineous fluid obtained from thoracentesis
• Fluid occupying one third of the involved lung, as shown on chest X-ray

MASSIVE HEMOTHORAX

Approximate blood loss
More than 2,000 ml

Signs and symptoms
• Dyspnea
• Tachypnea
• Hypotension
• Hypoxia
• Cyanosis
• Hypovolemic shock

Diagnostic findings
Same as those for moderate hemothorax, plus the following:
• fluid occupying half the involved lung, as shown on chest X-ray
• decreased hemoglobin
• absent breath sounds and dullness noted during percussion

REVIEWING CARE PRIORITIES

No matter what causes your patient's hemothorax, your first care priorities are to stabilize his condition, stop the bleeding, remove blood from the pleural cavity, and reexpand the involved lung. Exactly how you'll implement these goals depends on the hemothorax size.

Small-to-moderate hemothorax. This hemothorax type usually clears within 10 to 14 days. Your major responsibility is to watch for further bleeding. (However, the doctor may perform thoracentesis to treat a moderate hemothorax.)

Massive hemothorax. This condition requires chest-tube insertion to remove pleural cavity fluid. Be prepared to assist with the procedure.

As soon as the doctor confirms the diagnosis, he'll insert a chest tube into the fourth, fifth, or sixth intercostal space at the posterior axillary line. To prevent clot blockage, he'll probably use a large-bore tube and connect it to an underwater seal and suction. If the chest tube doesn't relieve the patient's condition, the doctor may perform a thoracotomy to control bleeding.

Nursing considerations. To care for the patient with a chest tube, take the steps outlined here:
• Explain all procedures to the patient to allay his fears.
• Administer oxygen, as ordered, by mask or nasal cannula.
• Give I.V. fluids and blood transfusions, as needed, to treat shock. Monitor arterial blood gas measurements frequently.
• Examine chest-tube drainage carefully, and document volume drained at least once an hour.
• Milk the chest tube every hour to keep it patent and free of clots. If the tube is warm and full of blood, and the fluid in the water seal bottle's rising rapidly, contact the doctor immediately. The patient may need immediate surgery.
• Monitor the patient's vital signs. Decreasing blood pressure and increasing pulse and respiratory rates may indicate shock. Also observe the patient for pallor and tachypnea.
• Apply medical antishock trousers (MAST suit), if ordered, to combat shock.
• Be ready to replace lost blood (when 2 to 3 units are drained from the pleural cavity). Autotransfusion may be used until compatible banked blood is available.

THORACOTOMY: INDICATIONS AND CONTRAINDICATIONS

Does your patient with a massive hemothorax need a thoracotomy? The doctor may perform this surgical procedure to control bleeding when:
• bloody drainage from the chest tube exceeds 400 ml/hour, or 200 ml/hour for 5 hours
• the hemothorax is massive
• the hemothorax increases, as shown by chest X-ray
• hypotension worsens or doesn't improve despite adequate blood replacement.

A thoracotomy's contraindicated when:
• blood pressure and pulse respond to blood replacement
• bloody drainage from the chest tube doesn't exceed 150 ml/hour after initial drainage
• chest X-ray shows reexpansion of the damaged lung, with no hemothorax recurrence on follow-up X-rays.

PENETRATING WOUNDS

COMPARING GUNSHOT AND STAB WOUNDS

Penetrating chest wounds rank second on the list of major chest trauma types that can alter respiratory status. (Blunt chest trauma heads the list.) Gunshot and stab wounds account for most penetrating injuries. But gunshot wounds are more serious, since they cause more rapid blood loss and severe lacerations, compro-

mising the patient's respiratory status immediately. And the bullet's ricochet effect often damages large body areas and multiple organs.

What's more, a gunshot wound's consequences are far less predictable than a stab wound's. A lucid and alert gunshot victim may suddenly be-

come disoriented or lose consciousness from rapid respiratory deterioration.

What does this mean to you? Obviously you'll have to work quickly and efficiently to assess the gunshot victim and take appropriate nursing actions. To discover how, read the following case history carefully.

CASE IN POINT

HOW TO INTERVENE

You're working the night shift in the emergency department when Joe Ross is admitted. A 43-year-old cab driver, Mr. Ross was robbed, then shot, by a passenger. He somehow managed to stay sufficiently alert and oriented to drive himself to the closest hospital—about 4 blocks away—and relate a cohesive account of the shooting.

As you inspect his chest, you pay particular attention to evidence of the entrance and exit wounds in Mr. Ross' chest. (Remember—even though a gunshot victim may appear stable, he's suffered a serious injury.) The small entrance wound in Mr. Ross' upper right chest at the second intercostal space over the midaxillary line is consistent with his description of the small-caliber weapon the holdup man used. Mr. Ross has no exit wounds, which means the bullet has probably lodged somewhere within his chest cavity. Surgery will be necessary to remove the bullet and repair damaged tissue.

Despite the wound's small size, Mr. Ross is in big trouble. The wound has produced an open pneumothorax—usually called a sucking chest wound—common in gunshot and stab victims. When you put your ear over the wound,

you hear a sucking sound when Mr. Ross breathes.

Because an open pneumothorax allows air into the chest cavity, the relative pressure in the pleural cavity changes from negative to positive. This places Mr. Ross at serious risk for collapsed lung, mediastinal shift, and impaired venous return. Fortunately, Mr. Ross hasn't developed these complications. But he's becoming increasingly dyspneic and complains of moderate pain in his left chest.

Intervention. Without rapid intervention, Mr. Ross' condition will deteriorate quickly. You cover the wound immediately with an occlusive petrolatum gauze dressing, which will let air seep out of the chest but prevent more air from entering.

Once you've applied the dressing, you watch closely for a developing tension pneumothorax. (At the first sign of this complication, you'd immediately remove the dressing to convert the tension pneumothorax back to an open pneumothorax, a less severe condition.)

To relieve Mr. Ross' respiratory distress, you give him oxygen by face mask at 6 liters/minute. Then you palpate and auscultate his

chest and abdomen to evaluate damage to adjacent organs and structures. You also auscultate for adventitious breath sounds, noting their location and quality.

Diagnosis. The doctor orders the following diagnostic tests:
• *Arterial blood gas (ABG) measurements.* These values reveal Mr. Ross' respiratory status.
• *Chest X-rays.* These tests help the doctor evaluate the injury and determine if chest tubes are necessary. Chest tubes can reestablish intrathoracic pressure and drain blood from the pleural cavity (in the case of a hemothorax). If chest tubes are inserted, order a follow-up X-ray to make sure the tubes are correctly positioned.
• *Complete blood count (CBC).* Hemoglobin, hematocrit, and differential may reveal severe blood loss. Arrange to have the patient's blood typed and cross-matched. Replace blood and fluids as necessary, and stay alert for hemorrhage.
• *EKG.* This test can reveal dysrhythmias—a leading cause of death in penetrating chest wound victims.
• Intake and output. The doctor will also instruct you to insert a Foley catheter to obtain specimens for urinalysis and to monitor urinary output.

HOW TO UNCOVER CLUES TO HELP PLAN YOUR PATIENT'S CARE

Before examining a penetrating wound victim, obtain as much information as possible from him about the incident. If he's unconscious or disoriented, question a family member, friend, or medical personnel, or speak to any police officers who were at the crime scene. The information you get may reveal important clues that help focus your assessment and tailor your care plan to the patient's immediate needs.

Since any gunshot or stabbing injury must be reported to the proper authorities, any information may be important legally. Make sure your nursing notes are thorough and accurate. Ask the victim of any penetrating chest injury the questions listed below.
• What type of gun or penetrating object caused the injury?
• What was the object's trajectory? For example, did it pass through a window or wall before striking you?
• From what range was the object propelled at you?
• Was the injury accidental or intentional?
• What type of gun or knife was used?
• If the weapon was a gun, do you know the caliber of the bullets?
• Were there any witnesses? If so, do you have their names, addresses, and telephone numbers?
• At what address did the incident occur?

The Law and You

HANDLING EVIDENCE: SOME IMPORTANT NURSING CONSIDERATIONS

Caring for a wound victim involves more than just attending to his physical needs. The legal implications of any shooting or stabbing require that you pay special attention to any evidence that may help authorities.

Most hospitals have written policies for handling evidence in cases of gunshot injury and other crimes. By following these guidelines precisely, you can supply authorities with a complete and accurate account of the injury, as well as preserve evidence in its original, untampered form:
• *The wound.* In your nursing notes, describe the initial appearance of the wound and related physical injuries, and note their location. State whether you saw burns or soot from the gun barrel. Also, record details about any treatments applied to the wound, such as cleansing or debriding. Be careful to describe only what you observe; don't make interpretations.
• *Clothing.* Search the patient's clothing carefully for bullets and other evidence. Whenever possible, keep clothing items intact. If you must cut clothing from the patient, cut around—not through—possible bullet holes or slashes.

After you've inspected clothing items, place them in a brown paper bag. (Don't use a plastic bag; it may develop condensation that could affect such clues as blood or soot.) On the bag, write the patient's name, date, and time. List all persons who handled the clothing.
• *Bullets, pellets, knives, frag-ments, and other specimens.* You may uncover specimens in your patient's clothing during assessment, or the doctor may retrieve them from the patient's body during surgery. In either case, place this potentially vital evidence in a sealed envelope labeled with the patient's name. Describe where, when, and how the specimens were found, including the date and exact time of the finding. Next, list the names of all persons who handled them. However, avoid excessive handling.

Also describe what, if anything, was done to the specimen; where it was kept; and how it was transported before it was turned over to authorities. Take every precaution not to alter the evidence in any way that might interfere with later identification.

Note: If your chest trauma victim has an object such as a knife impaled in his chest, don't remove it—for both legal and medical reasons. Removing it could destroy any fingerprints it may carry. And if the object's embedded in the heart, the lung, or a blood vessel, it could be helping to seal these structures. Sudden removal could cause profuse bleeding.

REFERENCES AND ACKNOWLEDGMENTS

Books

Anthony, Catherine P., and Thibodeau, Gary A. *Textbook of Anatomy and Physiology*, 10th ed. St. Louis: C.V. Mosby Co., 1979.

Assessment. Nurse's Reference Library. Springhouse, Pa.: Springhouse Corp., 1982.

Barber, Janet M., and Budassi, Susan A. *Mosby's Manual of Emergency Care: Practices and Procedures.* St. Louis: C.V. Mosby Co., 1979.

Barry, Jean. *Emergency Nursing.* New York: McGraw-Hill Book Co., 1977.

Borg, Nan, ed. *Core Curriculum for Critical Care Nurses.* American Association of Critical Care Nurses. Philadelphia: W.B. Saunders Co., 1981.

Brody, Jerome S. "Diseases of the Pleura, Mediastinum, Diaphragm, and Chest Wall," in *Cecil Textbook of Medicine*, 16th ed., vol. 1. Edited by Wyngaarden, James B., and Smith, Lloyd H., Jr. Philadelphia: W.B. Saunders Co., 1982.

Dealing with Emergencies. Nursing Photobook Series. Springhouse, Pa.: Springhouse Corp., 1980.

Diagnostics. Nurse's Reference Library. Springhouse, Pa.: Springhouse Corp., 1981.

Diseases. Nurse's Reference Library. Springhouse, Pa.: Springhouse Corp., 1981.

Drugs, 2nd ed. Nurse's Reference Library. Springhouse, Pa.: Springhouse Corp., 1984.

Duke University Hospital Nursing Services, ed. *Guidelines for Nursing Care: Process and Outcomes.* Philadelphia: J.B. Lippincott Co., 1983.

Ensuring Intensive Care. Nursing Photobook Series. Springhouse, Pa.: Springhouse Corp., 1981.

Fishman, Alfred P. *Pulmonary Diseases and Disorders*, 2 vols. New York: McGraw-Hill Book Co., 1979.

Giving Emergency Care Competently, 2nd ed. New Nursing Skillbook. Springhouse, Pa.: Springhouse Corp., 1983.

Guyton, Arthur C. *Textbook of Medical Physiology*, 6th ed. Philadelphia: W.B. Saunders Co., 1981.

Harper, Rosalind W. *A Guide to Respiratory Care: Physiology and Clinical Applications.* Philadelphia: J.B. Lippincott Co., 1982.

Hinshaw, H. Corwin, and Murray, John F. *Diseases of the Chest*, 4th ed. Philadelphia: W.B. Saunders Co., 1980.

Hirschmann, Jan V., and Murray, John F. "Pneumonia and Lung Abscess," in *Harrison's Principles of Internal Medicine*, 10th ed. Edited by Petersdorf, Robert G., et al. New York: McGraw-Hill Book Co., 1983.

Jones, Dorothy A., et al. *Medical-Surgical Nursing: A Conceptual Approach*, 2nd ed. New York: McGraw-Hill Book Co., 1982.

Keller, Colleen, and Solomon, Jacqueline. *Respiratory Nursing Care.* Englewood Cliffs, N.J.: Prentice-Hall, 1984.

Kenner, Cornelia V., et al. *Critical Care Nursing: Body-Mind-Spirit.* Boston: Little, Brown & Co., 1981.

Kinney, Marguerite, et al. *AACN's Clinical Reference for Critical Care Nursing.* New York: McGraw-Hill Book Co., 1981.

Kirsh, Marvin M., and Sloan, Herbert. *Blunt Chest Trauma: General Principles of Management.* Boston: Little, Brown & Co., 1977.

Phipps, Wilma J., et al. *Medical Surgical Nursing: Concepts and Clinical Practice*, 2nd ed. St. Louis: C.V. Mosby Co., 1983.

Providing Respiratory Care. Nursing Photobook Series. Springhouse, Pa.: Springhouse Corp., 1983.

Sexton, Dorothy L. *Chronic Obstructive Pulmonary Disease: Care of the Child and Adult.* St. Louis: C.V. Mosby Co., 1981.

Shapiro, Barry A., et al. *Clinical Application of Respiratory Care*, 2nd ed. Chicago: Year Book Medical Pubs., 1979.

Shoemaker, William C., et al. *Textbook of Critical Care.* Philadelphia: W.B. Saunders Co., 1984.

Wade, Jacqueline F. *Comprehensive Respiratory Care: Physiology and Technique*, 3rd ed. St. Louis: C.V. Mosby Co., 1982.

West, John B. *Respiratory Physiology: The Essentials*, 2nd ed. Baltimore: Williams & Wilkins Co., 1979.

Periodicals

Boettger, M.L. ''Scuba Diving Emergencies: Pulmonary Overpressure Accidents and Decompression Sickness,'' *Annals of Emergency Medicine* 12(9):563-67, September 1983.

Bullas, J.B. ''Fibrinolytic Therapy: Nursing Implications,'' *Critical Care Nurse* 1:43-46, November/December 1981.

Dossey, B., and Passons, J.M. ''Pulmonary Embolism: Preventing It, Treating It,'' *Nursing81* 11:26-33, March 1981.

Griffin, J.P. ''Nursing Care of Patients on High-Frequency Jet Ventilation,'' *Critical Care Nurse* 4:25-28, November/December 1981.

Griffin, J.P., and Carlon, G.C. ''Medical and Nursing Implications of High-Frequency Jet Ventilation,''·*Heart and Lung* 13(3):250-54, May 1984.

Hamer, S.S., and Lemberg, L. ''A Complication Commonly Overlooked... Acute Pulmonary Embolism,'' *Heart and Lung,* 11(6):588-92, November/December 1982.

Hoyt, K.S. ''Chest Trauma,'' *Nursing83* 13(5):34-41, May 1983.

Pinnyei, M.K. ''Management of Gunshot Injuries,'' *Dimensions of Critical Care Nursing* 2(6):344-52, November/December 1983.

Sasahara, A.A., et al. ''Pulmonary Thromboembolism. Diagnosis and Treatment,'' *Journal of the American Medical Association* 249(21): 2945-50, June 3, 1983.

Sharma, G.V., et al. ''Drug Therapy: Thrombolytic Therapy,'' *New England Journal of Medicine* 306(21):1268-76, May 27, 1982.

Sharma, G.V., et al. ''Pulmonary Embolism,'' *Cardiovascular Clinician* 13(2):155-70, 1983.

Sonnenblick, M., et al. ''Body Positional Effect on Gas Exchange in Unilateral Pleural Effusion,'' *Chest: The Cardiopulmonary Journal* 83(5):784-86, May 1983.

Unger, K. ''Pulmonary Embolism,'' *American Family Practice* 26(4):192-98, 1982.

Williams, M.H. ''Pulmonary Embolism,'' *Emergency Medicine* 14:84-93, June 15, 1982.

We'd like to thank the following companies for their help with this book:

ARMSTRONG INDUSTRIES, INC.
Northbrook, Ill.

BECTON, DICKSON AND CO.
Oxnard, Calif.

CHESEBROUGH–POND'S INC.
Greenwich, Conn.

LAERDAL MEDICAL CORPORATION
Armonk, N.Y.

LYNE–NICHOLSON, INC.
Needham Heights, Mass.

SHILEY, INC.
Irvine, Calif.

SUTTERBIOMEDICAL INC.
San Diego, Calif.

TAMPA TRACINGS
Tarpon Springs, Fla.

We'd also like to thank the staffs of:

MEMORIAL HOSPITAL, ROXBOROUGH
Philadelphia
Max Tugendreich, RRT
Acting Director,
Respiratory Therapy

NATIONAL INSTITUTES OF HEALTH—
NATIONAL HEART, LUNG, AND BLOOD INSTITUTE
Bethesda, Md.

PHILADELPHIA HEALTH MANAGEMENT CORP.
Philadelphia
John McCartney
Program Specialist

TEMPLE UNIVERSITY MEDICAL SCIENCES CENTER
Philadelphia
Virginia D. Elsenhans, RN, MEd, CNP
Medical Group Practices

UNIVERSITY OF PENNSYLVANIA
Philadelphia
Joyce P. Griffin, RN, MSN, CCRN
Instructor, School of Nursing

INDEX

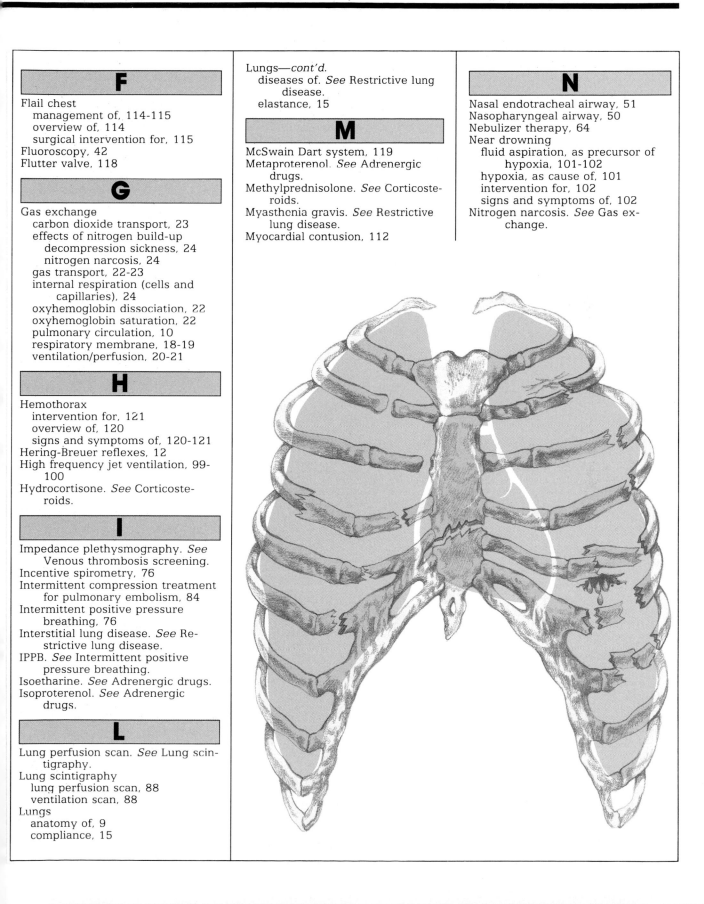

INDEX

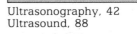
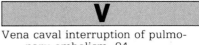